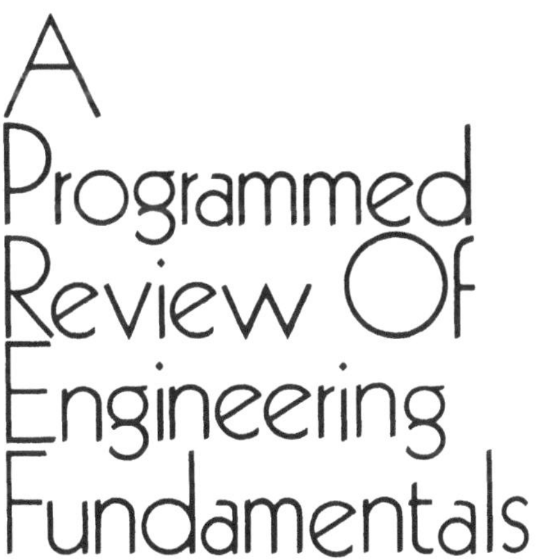
A
Programmed
Review Of
Engineering
Fundamentals

A Programmed Review Of Engineering Fundamentals

ALLEN J. BALDWIN, P.E.
KAREN M. HESS, Ph.D.

VNR Springer Science+Business Media, LLC

Originally published by Van Nostrand Reinhold Inc., 1978
MyCopy version of the original edition 1978

DOI 10.1007/978-1-4757-1223-0

15 14 13 12 11 10 9 8 7 6 5 4 3 2 1

Library of Congress Cataloging in Publication Data

Baldwin, Allen J.
A programmed review of engineering fundamentals.

Includes index.
1. Engineering–Programmed instruction.
2. Engineering–Examinations, questions, etc.
I. Hess, Karen M., 1939- joint author. II. Title.
TA159.B34 620'.007'7 78-1823
www.springer.com/mycopy

Preface

Engineering registration is accelerating at a pace unequalled since institution of registration laws in the 1920s and 1930s. This phenomenon is not due to an easing of entrance requirements, since only vestiges of "grandfathering" and eminence exist in most states. Nor is it due to a lessening in the difficulty of the registration examinations. In fact, it is generally agreed that the Engineering Fundamentals Examination has significantly increased in difficulty over the last fifteen years.

Why then the increased interest in registration among practicing engineers?

Historically the professional engineer has been in private practice offering consulting services directly to the public. Registration laws were passed to protect the public from incompetent, untrained practioners in any engineering area. However, the registration laws go beyond establishing an individual's credentials. One reason for the new interest in engineering registration is the proliferation of new activity areas such as pollution control and energy conservation where the public is keenly aware of and insistent upon quality technological inputs.

A second reason for the increased interest in registration also relates to the consumer movement. Registration laws in most states do *not* apply to manufacturers. This so-called industry exemption is under attack by consumers who are concerned about unsafe products designed by anonymous employees of a corporation subject to no public control over their level of competence. Because of this consumer concern, many large firms are strongly encouraging their engineers to become registered so that in any possible lawsuit involving a firm its employees can appear in court as professionals.

Further, engineers themselves are becoming more aware that licensure is a necessary requirement of a profession, a key factor in the control *of* the profession *by* the profession. Without licensure, such other control mechanisms as school accreditation, entrance requirements, and continuing education are ineffective: anyone can practice without conforming to these controls.

Finally, reciprocity among states has become a reality. In the past each state gave its own examination; there was little or no reciprocity. Now, however, the National Council of Engineering Examiners (NCEE) has instituted a national examination in virtually all states. This book is designed as a study aid for the NCEE Engineering Fundamentals Examination.

Prerequisites for the Examination

The prerequisite for admission to the Engineering Fundamentals Examination is usually graduation from an accredited engineering college. Application is made to the local state board of registration. The exams are usually given twice yearly, in November and April; the fee varies from state to state.

The Engineering Fundamentals Examination

The examination is an open-book, eight-hour, written exam given in two four-hour parts.

Part I is usually open-book, multiple-choice. The examinee answers as many questions as he can from the following distribution.

Mathematics	15%
Nucleonics and wave phenomena	3%
Chemistry	9%
Statics	9%
Dynamics	9%
Mechanics of materials	9%
Fluid mechanics	9%
Thermodynamics	12%
Electrical theory	12%
Materials science	5%
Economics	8%

Part II is usually open-book problem solving. It consists of three problems each in seven subjects:

Dynamics
Mechanics of materials
Thermodynamics
Electrical theory
Statics
Fluid mechanics
Economics analysis

The Part II problems consist of introductory information about a problem situation, followed by ten multiple choice questions concerning the problem. Typically the applicant selects five of the twenty-one problems in accordance with the following rules:

1. The five problems must be distributed among at least four subjects.
2. Not more than one problem can be selected in economics.

Each state can and often does change the above rules slightly. The examinee should carefully study the rules in effect at the time and place of the examination. The rules listed above are meant as guidelines for preparing to take the exam.

This Text

This text had its inception in a professional society study conducted in 1969 to find ways to help and encourage engineers to become registered. It became clear that a graduating senior from an accredited school usually had little difficulty passing the Engineering Fundamentals Examination, but approximately half of those taking the examination had been away from the academic environment for several years. For this mature engineer, little help was available. As a result, a refresher course was initiated to assist the engineer with several years of experience prepare for the fundamentals examination.

This text is an outgrowth of the experience gained from the refresher course from 1969 to the present. The text has been prepared to closely simulate the multiple-choice questions in the national examination. The questions are similar in scope and content to those in both Parts I and II of the exam.

Each chapter presents a brief summary of the chapter's content, followed by basic textual material related to specific concepts and principles. The key concepts, boxed for clarity, are followed by examples and one or two application problems for you to work. The answers to the problems are given immediately after each problem, providing you with an immediate indication of your understanding of each concept.

How to Use This Book

Work through the book in sequence. However, if some material in the first section is too basic, skip it. For most the basic drill in mathematics pays off in later chapters.

Use your own reference tables and charts. These have purposely been omitted from this text as you should have access to and be familiar with basic reference tables and charts during the examination if it is open-book in your state.

Use your reference books to look up any terms and definitions which you do not understand in this text. All terms and definitions cannot be contained in a single text. However, the basic principles you will need to pass the exam are included.

Do *not* skip the "afternoon set" problems presented at the end of each chapter in the second section. These problems are typical of those contained in Part II of the exam and constitute one-half of the exam.

Do not elect in advance to skip certain subjects. This will limit your options when you take the exam. You may be an electrical engineer, but the exam may contain some very easy questions in thermodynamics which you should answer.

Always check you answers with those given. Certain mistakes are commonly made on some problems. In these cases the wrong answer is included among the choices. You will then be led to believe you have the right answer when, in fact, you are wrong. If this happens to you, go back to see where you have made your error and why the right answer is right.

ALLEN J. BALDWIN, P.E.
KAREN M. HESS, PH.D.

Contents

A Programmed Review Of Engineering Fundamentals

Part I Mathematics and Science

Part I of this book reviews the basic mathematics and science principles covered in the morning session of the National Engineering Fundamentals Examination. Since the morning session problems are in multiple-choice format, this book also presents the problems in multiple-choice format.

1 Algebra

Discussion of and problems related to conversion, factoring, quadratic equations, combining exponents, scientific notation, simultaneous equations, determinants, simultaneous equations, logarithms, and laws of logarithms.

A. DEFINITION

Algebra provides tools for converting a problem from the English language into mathematical language. Thus, it is more powerful than ordinary arithmetic. The basic tool of algebra is the *equation*. An equation is a statement of fact, a truism. The equal sign (=) in algebra corresponds to the word *is* in the English language.

The English word *is* is equivalent to the algebraic equal sign (=).

Example

The English phrase, "The engine produces 50 horsepower" is written algebraically as Hp = 50.

PROBLEMS

1. The Greek mathematician Euclid, lacking algebra, said in 300 B.C.: "The circumference of a circle is 3.141592 times its diameter." State this truism in the language of algebra:

____

2. Sir Isaac Newton said: "The acceleration of a body is proportional to the force acting on it and inversely proportional to its mass." What is the algebraic equation? (Circle the letter of the correct response.)

   a. $F = ma$. b. $a \propto F/m$. c. $S = \frac{1}{2}at^2$. d. $F \propto am$. e. $a \propto Fm$.

   Check your answers with those which follow.

Answers

1. (Circumference) = (3.141592) × (Diameter) OR $C = \pi D$.
   The word *is* is equivalent to =. The word *times* is equivalent to ×.
2. b.
   The word *proportional* is the same as the word *is* if the units of the variables are correct. You may want to check the dictionary for the meaning of "inversely proportional."

B. CONVERSION–INDEPENDENT AND DEPENDENT VARIABLES

The first step in solving a problem using algebra is to *convert* the nouns (things) in the problem into algebraic symbols. The convention is to use the letters in the first half of the alphabet (a, b, c, etc.) for things that have *known* values. These are called *independent variables* because their values are fixed and not influenced by the problem. The letters in the last half of the alphabet (u, v, w, x, y, z) are reserved for things that have *unknown* values. These are *dependent variables* because their values are determined by the problem itself.

> *Independent variables* are the values given in the problem–knowns.
> *Dependent variables* are controlled by the circumstances of the problem–unknowns.

Example

The sum of two numbers is 18. One number is double the other. The sum is an independent variable: $a = 18$. The numbers are dependent variables: $x = ?$ $2x = ?$

The equation relating the variables is:

$$x + 2x = a$$

$$3x = 18$$

$$x = 18/3.$$

The numbers are:

$$x = 6$$

$$2x = 12.$$

PROBLEMS

1. °F = 9/5°C + 32.
   The Celsius temperature is 10° (independent variable).
   What is the Fahrenheit temperature (dependent variable)?

   a. -40°F. b. 128°F. c. 50°F. d. 100°F. e. -459°F.

2. The velocity of car A is 50 mph, north.
   The velocity of car B is 60 mph, south.
   A is 165 miles south of B. How long until they meet?

   a. 1 hr 25 min. b. 1 hr. c. 2 hrs. d. 1 hr 30 min. e. 2 hrs 20 min.

   Check your answers with those which follow.

Answers

1. c.
2. d.
   If your answers are not correct, review the definition of *algebra*, p. 3.

C. FACTORING

Manipulation such as that in the previous problems is subject to rules based on the form of the equation. The first step in solving a problem is to rearrange the equation into its simplest form. This is called *factoring*.

> *Forms of Equations:*
> Linear: $x = a$
> Quadratic: $x^2 = b$
> nth-degree polynomial: $x^n = c$
> General form of a third degree polynomial
> $$c_3x^3 + c_2x^2 + c_1x^1 + c_0x^0 = 0$$

Example

To simplify the equation $ax + bx = c$:
combine the coefficients of x: $x(a + b) = c$;
divide both sides by $(a + b)$:

$$x\frac{(a+b)}{(a+b)} = \frac{c}{(a+b)}.$$

Therefore, the simplest form of the linear equation is

$$x = \frac{c}{a+b}.$$

PROBLEMS

1. Simplify the following equation:

$$4x + 8x^2 + 12x^3 = 0.$$

---

2. Simplify the following equation:

$$x^4 - xy^3 - x^3y + y^4 = 0.$$

Check your answers with those which follow.

Answers

1. $4x(1 + 2x + 3x^2) = 0.$
   The simplification accomplished here consists of reducing the degree of the terms. In other words, the highest exponent appearing is reduced from 3 to 2.
2. $(x - y)^2(x^2 + xy + y^2) = 0.$
   If you had difficulty with this simplification, refer to a table of factoring formulas in an algebra text. Reducing the degree of this equation from 4 to 2 means we can treat it as a quadratic. The advantages of working with quadratics will be covered next.

D. QUADRATIC EQUATIONS

A quadratic equation is a second-degree polynomial. In other words, the highest exponent is 2. There is a powerful formula for solving quadratic equations. If a quadratic equation is in the form:

$$ax^2 + bx + c = 0,$$

then:

$$\boxed{x = \frac{-b \pm \sqrt{b^2 - 4ac}}{2a}.}$$

Example

In the equation $x^2 = 9$, the coefficients a, b, and c have the following values:

$$a = 1$$

$$b = 0$$

$$c = -9$$

and the solution is:

$$x = \frac{-0 \pm \sqrt{0^2 - (4)(1)(-9)}}{(2)(1)}$$

$$= \frac{-0 \pm \sqrt{36}}{2}$$

$$= \pm 3.$$

The ± sign indicates that there are two solutions, both of which are correct. Note that $(3)^2 = 9$ and $(-3)^2 = 9$. In general, for any polynomial the number of solutions equals the degree of the polynomial.

PROBLEMS

1. $\sqrt{x^2 + 6x} = x + \sqrt{2x}$. What are the values of x?

   ____

2. $3x^2 - 6x + 4 = 0$; $x =$

   a. 4.46, 2.46. b. $1 \pm \frac{\sqrt{-12}}{6}$ c. $1 \pm \frac{\sqrt{-12}}{6}$ d. $2 \pm \sqrt{-16}$. e. 3.46, 1.46.

3. Rationalize the number $\frac{2 + i}{4 + i3}$.

   a. $\frac{(2 + i)(4 + i3)}{25}$. b. $\frac{11 - 2i}{25}$. c. $\frac{11 + 2i}{25}$. d. $\frac{8 + 3i}{4 + 3i}$. e. $\frac{1}{2} - \frac{i}{3}$.

4. A ball is thrown straight up. Its position as a function of time is: $S = 96t - 16t^2$. What is the maximum height reached? $S =$

   a. 64 ft. b. 288 ft. c. 144 ft. d. 164 ft. e. 128 ft.

   Check your answers.

Answers

1. $x = 0, x = 2$.
   You must square both sides of the equation twice to eliminate the radicals ($\sqrt{\ }$) before applying the quadratic formula.
2. b.
   The term $\sqrt{-12}$ is called an imaginary term because there is no real number which can be squared to yield -12. In general, you will seldom see imaginary answers in practical problems. A combination of real and imaginary terms is called a complex number. The com-

plex roots of this equation are:

$$x = 1 + i2 \quad \text{and} \quad x = 1 - i2$$

where $i = \sqrt{-1}$.

3. b.
   You may want to look up a definition of "rationalize" if you had difficulty with this problem.
4. c.
   Set up the quadratic formula with $c = s$. When s is low the term under the radical is positive. But as s increases, the term becomes negative. An imaginary solution means the ball never gets that high. The maximum height corresponds to the distance at which the term under the radical goes from positive to negative, i.e., the term equals 0.

E. COMBINING EXPONENTS

Manipulations sometimes involve operations whereby exponents must be combined. Note that in the laws of exponents presented below the arithmetic operation on the exponent is one order less than on the base. In other words, if the bases are multiplied, the exponents are added.

Laws of Exponents:
$(a^p)(a^g) = a^{(p+g)}$
$(a^p)^g = a^{pg}$
$a^p/a^g = a^{(p-g)}$
$(ab)^p = a^p b^p$
$a^{m/n} = \sqrt[n]{a^m}$
$a^{-m/n} = \sqrt[n]{1/a^m}$
$a^0 = 1.$

Example

$$(x^2)(x^3) = x^5.$$

PROBLEMS

1. Evaluate: $(\frac{1}{4})^{3/2}$.

   a. $\frac{1}{2}$. b. $\frac{3}{16}$. c. $\frac{3}{8}$. d. $\frac{1}{6}$. e. $\frac{1}{8}$.

2. Evaluate: $(-8)^{-2/3} \times (2)^2$.

   a. $-16^{1/3}$. b. 4. c. 1. d. $\frac{1}{16}$. e. $6^{4/3}$.

   Check your answers.

Answers

1. e.
2. c.
   If you had difficulty with these problems, review the laws of exponents, p. 8.

F. SCIENTIFIC NOTATION

Scientific notation is a tool for placing the decimal point in a number in terms of powers of 10. Manipulations can then be done using the laws of exponents.

$(N)(10)^x$ means x zeros after N.
$(N)(10)^{-x}$ means x zeros after the decimal point.

Examples

$$24{,}000 = 24 \times 10^3$$

$$0.0016 = 16 \times 10^{-4}$$

PROBLEM

Using scientific notation, evaluate:

$$\sqrt[3]{\frac{(0.004)^4 (0.0036)^1}{(120{,}000)^2}}$$

a. 4×10^{-8}. b. 0.0004. c. 12×10^{-6}. d. 4×10^{-24}. e. 2×10^{-8}.

Check your answer.

Answer

a.

G. SIMULTANEOUS EQUATIONS

So far all the examples of equations presented have involved only one unknown. An example of an equation containing two unknowns is $x + y = 5$. This equation cannot be solved for specific values of x and y since a whole family of values will satisfy the equation:

x	y
1	4
2	3
3	2
4	1

All of these values satisfy $x + y = 5$. But, suppose we have another equation which is also true in this case: $x - y = 1$. Only the solution $x = 3$, $y = 2$ is a common solution to both of these equations. The two equations are called *simultaneous equations* because they are both true at the same time (simultaneously).

> For a specific solution there must be as many simultaneous equations as there are unknowns.

Example

An airplane flies from St. Louis to Chicago, a distance of 500 miles, in 2 hours against the wind. Returning the trip takes 1.5 hours. What is the ground speed of the plane? What is the wind velocity?

$$x = \text{ground speed}$$

$$y = \text{wind velocity}$$

1. $$2(x - y) = 500$$

2. $$1.5(x + y) = 500$$

Rearranging 1:

$$x = 250 + y.$$

Substituting in 2:

$$1.5(250 + y + y) = 500.$$

$$y = 41.7 \text{ wind velocity}$$

$$x = 250 + 41.7$$

$$= 291.7 \text{ ground speed}$$

PROBLEMS

1. What are the dimensions of a rectangle with an area of 150 ft^2 and a perimeter of 50 ft?

___

2. You have \$1.30 in change. There are 3 dimes for every quarter and 2 more nickles than there are quarters. Exactly what coins do you have?

Check your answers.

Answers

1. 10 ft X 15 ft.
Set up two simultaneous equations to algebraically state the above two facts.
2. 4 nickles, 2 quarters, and 6 dimes.
This problem requires three simultaneous equations. If you like, use determinants covered in the following section to rework it.

H. DETERMINANTS

There is a systematic way of putting numbers in an array resulting in what is called a *determinant.* A three-by-three determinant is defined as follows:

$$\begin{vmatrix} a_1 & b_1 & c_1 \\ a_2 & b_2 & c_2 \\ a_3 & b_3 & c_3 \end{vmatrix} = a_1b_2c_3 + b_1c_2a_3 + c_1a_2b_3 - c_1b_2a_3 - a_1c_2b_3 - b_1a_2c_3$$

Example

Evaluate the determinant:

$$\begin{vmatrix} 2 & 6 \\ 3 & 4 \end{vmatrix} = (2)(4) - (6)(3)$$

$$= -10$$

PROBLEM

Evaluate the determinant:

$$\begin{vmatrix} 1 & 3 & 0 \\ 0 & 1 & 1 \\ 12 & 2 & 4 \end{vmatrix}$$

Check your answer.

Answer

38.

I. DETERMINANTS AND SIMULTANEOUS EQUATIONS

Determinants can be used to solve systems of simultaneous equations; n simultaneous equations will require $n \times n$ determinants. Below is the rule for a system of three simultaneous equations.

$$a_1x + b_1y + c_1z = d_1$$
$$a_2x + b_2y + c_2z = d_2$$
$$a_3x + b_3y + c_3z = d_3.$$
$$x = \frac{\begin{vmatrix} d_1 & b_1 & c_1 \\ d_2 & b_2 & c_2 \\ d_3 & b_3 & c_3 \end{vmatrix}}{\begin{vmatrix} a_1 & b_1 & c_1 \\ a_2 & b_2 & c_2 \\ a_3 & b_3 & c_3 \end{vmatrix}}.$$

Example

$2x + 3y = 4.$
$x + 2y = 1.$

$$x = \frac{\begin{vmatrix} 4 & 3 \\ 1 & 2 \end{vmatrix}}{\begin{vmatrix} 2 & 3 \\ 1 & 2 \end{vmatrix}} = \frac{8 - 3}{4 - 3} = 5, \qquad y = \frac{\begin{vmatrix} 2 & 4 \\ 1 & 1 \end{vmatrix}}{\begin{vmatrix} 2 & 3 \\ 1 & 2 \end{vmatrix}} = \frac{2 - 4}{4 - 3} = -2.$$

PROBLEM

Solve the following three simultaneous equations for x and z:

$$x + 2y - z = -3$$
$$3x + y + z = 4$$
$$x - y + 2z = 6$$

Check your answer.

Answer

$x = 1, z = 2.$
If you had difficulty with this problem, look for the patterns in the definition.

J. LOGARITHMS

A transcendental function is one that has been arbitrarily derived to do a particular job. One such transcendental function is the *logarithm* (log) which is arbitrarily defined as follows:

$$\begin{array}{|lll|}\hline \text{If} & b^x & = N \\ \text{then} & x & = \log_b N \\ \hline\end{array}$$

b is called the base of the logarithm and is commonly taken as 10 (common) or e (natural or Napierian), where $e = 2.71828$. Conventionally, the term log means $\log_{10}$ and ln means $\log_e$.

Example

$$10^3 = 1000.$$

Therefore $\log_{10} 1000 = 3$.

PROBLEMS

1. In chemistry

$$p\text{H} = \log \frac{1}{[\text{H}]}.$$

What is the value of [H] if the $p\text{H} = 8$? [H] =

a. 8^{10}. b. 10^8. c. 10^{-8}. d. 8×10^{-2}. e. $\frac{1}{10}^{-8}$.

2. If $y = e^x$, $\ln y =$

a. x. b. $\log_e 4$. c. 10^x. d. 1. e. y^{10}.

Check your answers.

Answers

1. c.
2. a.

If you had difficulty with these problems, review the definition of logarithm given above.

K. LAWS OF LOGARITHMS

The advantage of using logarithms is that the arithmetic in a given operation can be simplified by using the laws of logarithms:

$$\log (M)(N) = \log M + \log N$$

$$\log \frac{(M)}{(N)} = \log M - \log N$$

$$\log (M)^p = p \log M$$

Note that in each case the arithmetic level was reduced. Multiplication became addition, division became subtraction, and the exponent was reduced to a multiplication.

The examples which follow will be carried out using common logarithms to the base 10. The common logarithm is in two parts:

1. The characteristic is to the left of the decimal point.
2. The mantissa is to the right of the decimal point.

Characteristic for number greater than 1: characteristic is positive and is one less than the number of digits before the decimal point.

Characteristic for number less than 1: characteristic is negative and is one more than the number of zeros following the decimal point.

The mantissa is found by referring to a table of common logarithms.

Examples

1. The log of 46.38 = 1.6663.
2. The log of 0.04638 = $\bar{2}.6663$. (NOTE: Only the characteristic is negative; the mantissa is always positive.)
3. Logarithms are particularly useful in working with non-integer exponents.
   To evaluate $(0.9)^{0.31}$,

$$\log (0.9)^{0.31} = 0.31 \log 0.9$$
$$= (0.31)(\bar{1}.9542)$$
$$= \bar{1}.9858$$

Remember, the characteristic is negative; the mantissa is positive.
Now take the antilog:

$$\log N = \bar{1}.9858$$
$$N = .9678$$

PROBLEMS

1. $(6.12)^{1/20} =$

   a. 1.090. b. 1.105. c. 1.050. d. 1.095. e. 1.085.

2. $e^{(x)(\ln y)} =$

   a. $\dfrac{\ln x}{\log 10}$. b. x^y. c. $\log_{10} e^x$. d. $\dfrac{e^x - e^{-x}}{e^x + e^{-x}}$. e. y^x.

Check your answers.

Answers

1. d.
   You should use a calculator or four-place log tables for accuracy.
2. e.
   Apply the basic definition of a logarithm.

2 Probability

Discussion of and problems related to joint probability, mutually exclusive events, repeated trials, binomial distribution, and normal distribution.

A. DEFINITION

The *probability* of an event occurring is the numerical ratio of the total number of ways an event can occur to the total possible outcomes. For example, in a toss of a die the probability of a five is 1/6, since there is only one way a five can result and there are six possible outcomes.

This definition holds for dichotomous events which are characterized by either success or failure with no middle ground. Real-life events can be dichotomized by carefully defining success. For example, in shooting a rifle success could be hitting the bull's eye or it could be simply hitting the target. For either case, failure would be defined as all other possible outcomes.

$$\boxed{P = \frac{N_{\text{success}}}{N_{\text{total}}} = 1 - \frac{N_{\text{failure}}}{N_{\text{total}}}.}$$

Example

The probability of drawing a Jack out of a deck of cards is

$$P(\text{Jack}) = 4/52,$$

while the probability of a Jack of Clubs is

$$P(\text{Jack of Clubs}) = 1/52.$$

PROBLEM

Three coins are tossed. What is the probability that all three will be heads?

a. 1/4.
b. 1/9.
c. 1/3.
d. 1/6.
e. 1/8.

Check your answer.

Answer

e.
To solve this problem, carefully list the possible outcomes, bearing in mind that a head for coin 1 and tails for 2 and 3 (*HTT*) is a different outcome than (*THT*) or (*TTH*). Another way of conceptualizing this problem will be covered in the next section.

B. JOINT PROBABILITY

Probability problems become complex only when events are put together in what is termed a *probability set*. The first probability set to be covered is one where the events are related by a *joint probability*. There are two such relationships: independent events and dependent events.

Independent Events

The repeated tosses of a coin are independent, since the outcome of the nth toss is independent of all previous tosses. The probability of two heads in a row is

$$P(HH) = (1/2)(1/2) = 1/4.$$

Joint probabilities are always the product of all individual event probabilities. Joint probabilities stated in English always contain or imply the word *and*. In the case above, "two heads in a row" can be restated as "a head on the first toss *and* a head on the second toss."

Dependent Events

Dependent events differ only in that the event probability on the nth trial depends on previous outcomes. The probability of drawing two Aces from a deck of cards is

$$(4/52)(3/51) = 12/2652.$$

In the second draw there are only 3 Aces left and only 51 cards. This is called "drawing without replacement." If we had replaced the first card these two events would be independent. Note the multiplication as in the case of independent events. Also, note the importance of the word *and* in the statement of the problem.

Summary

Joint probabilities are the probability of success on trial 1 *and* the probability of success on trial 2 *and* trial 3, etc.

$$\boxed{P(AB) = P(A) \times P(B).}$$

Example

In a gambling game you will win \$1.60 if you can toss a coin 3 times and get all heads. How much would you be willing to pay to play this game?

You would pay no more than the "expected value" of your winnings:

$$\text{Expected Value} = [P(\text{win})]\,(\text{winnings})$$

$$P(\text{win}) = P(HHH) = (1/2)(1/2)(1/2) = 1/8$$

$$\text{Expected Value} = (1/8)(\$1.60) = 20¢.$$

PROBLEM

The chance of the valves and piston rings in an automobile lasting 60,000 miles is 0.9. There is a 0.02 chance that the auto will need a valve job before this time. What is the chance that the rings will last 60,000 miles?

a. 0.92.
b. 0.88.
c. 0.96.
d. 0.91.
e. 0.18.

Check your answer.

Answer

a.

$$P(\text{rings}) \div P(\text{valves}) = 0.918.$$

C. MUTUALLY EXCLUSIVE EVENTS

A probability set where the occurrence of one event precludes the occurrence of another is made up of *mutually exclusive events.* In the tossing of a coin there are two mutually exclusive outcomes, a head and a tail. A probability set could be the probability of a head or a tail on a single toss. Here the probability is obviously one, but it is also the sum of the mutually exclusive events: (1/2) + (1/2). In this case the probability set is an exhaustive set since it contains all mutually exclusive possibilities. The sum of probabilities in an exhaustive set total unity.

Also note the importance of the word *or*. Mutually exclusive events are always characterized by an *or* statement. For example, what is the probability of tossing two coins and getting a head and a tail? The outcomes are:

Coin 1	*Coin 2*	*Probability*
H	H	1/4
H	T	1/4
T	H	1/4
T	T	1/4

There are two mutually exclusive ways of getting a head and a tail: coin 1 is a head and coin 2 is a tail OR coin 1 is a tail and coin 2 is a head.

$$P(HT \text{ or } TH) = P(HT) + P(TH) = (1/4) + (1/4) = 1/2.$$

Example

One urn contains 4 white balls and 2 black balls. A second urn contains 3 white balls and 5 black balls. What is the probability of drawing two balls, one from each urn, one white and one black?

This can happen in two mutually exclusive ways:

The first ball is white and the second is black.

OR

The first ball is black and the second is white.

$$P(A) = (4/6)(5/8) = 5/12$$

$$P(B) = (2/6)(3/8) = 1/8$$

$$P(A \text{ or } B) = (5/12) + (1/8) = 13/24.$$

PROBLEMS

1. What is the probability of drawing an Ace, a King, and a Queen in three draws from a deck of cards?

   a. 192/140,608.
   b. 384/132,600.
   c. 64/132,600.
   d. 384/140,608.
   e. 192/132,600.

2. An engineer feels his chances of passing each of the two engineering examinations is 0.5.

He will be allowed to take each exam up to three times. What is the probability that this man will become a registered professional engineer?

a. 0.67.
b. 0.25.
c. 0.96.
d. 0.62.
e. 0.77.

Check your answers.

Answers

1. b.
   There are six mutually exclusive ways you can draw an Ace, a King, and a Queen—count them. The three draws are also dependent events.
2. e.

D. REPEATED TRIALS

For practical problems it is common for the number of repeated trials to be so large that the foregoing methods are cumbersome. In such cases the repeated trials formula is helpful.

Repeated trials: Probability of an event happening exactly r times in n trials:

$$P(r,n) = \frac{n!}{r!(n-r)!} p^r(1-p)^{n-r}.$$

Factorial notation:

$$5! = 5 \times 4 \times 3 \times 2 \times 1$$

$$0! = 1 \text{ by definition.}$$

(Note the results if we were to calculate the probability of exactly no successes in n trials.)

The above formula is also useful in calculating the probability of "at least" n successes in n trials.

Example

If a coin is tossed 6 times, what is the probability of getting at least 3 heads?

$$P(\text{exactly 3 heads}) = \frac{6!}{3!3!}(1/2)^3(1/2)^3 = 20(1/2)^6$$

$$P(\text{exactly 4 heads}) = \frac{6!}{4!2!}(1/2)^4(1/2)^2$$
$$= 15(1/2)^6$$
$$P(\text{exactly 5 heads}) = \frac{6!}{5!1!}(1/2)^6 = 6(1/2)^6$$
$$P(\text{exactly 6 heads}) = \frac{6!}{6!}(1/2)^6 = (1/2)^6.$$

These are four mutually exclusive events.

$$P(\text{at least 3}) = (20 + 15 + 6 + 1)(1/2)^6$$
$$= 21/32.$$

PROBLEM

What is the chance of declaring that a lot of a product has a quality level of 0.9 or better based on a sample of 10 if the quality level is really 0.8?

a. 3.0×10^{-2}.
b. 0.2×10^{-1}.
c. 3.8×10^{-1}.
d. 1.9×10^{-1}.
e. 6.3×10^{-1}.

Check your answer.

Answer

c.
Repeated trials adding $P(9,10) + P(10,10)$ given $p = 0.8$.

E. BINOMIAL DISTRIBUTION

A probability distribution is a complete probability set with all possible combinations in tabular form. In the case of dichotomous events such as we have been discussing, such a probability set is called a *binomial distribution*. The binomial distribution deals with discrete measurements which are dichotomous.

> The *binomial distribution* deals with discrete or dichotomous events.

Example

A missile manufacturer claims that his product has a reliability of 0.90. The Air Force tests 5 of his missiles by firing them and they all work. What conclusions can be drawn?

This is the same as drawing 5 balls from an urn with 90 white balls and 10 black balls:

$$P(5,5) = \frac{5!}{5!0!}(0.9)^5(0.1)^0 = 0.590$$

$$P(4,5) \qquad = 0.328$$

$$P(3,5) \qquad = 0.073$$

$$P(2,5) \qquad = 0.008$$

etc.

The above probabilities indicate the likelihood of separate outcomes. If the reliability is 0.90, the most likely outcome is 5 successes, but note that there is also a significant (0.328) chance of only 4 successes.

The table developed in the above problem is a discrete distribution commonly known as the binomial distribution. Graphically, it could be illustrated as follows:

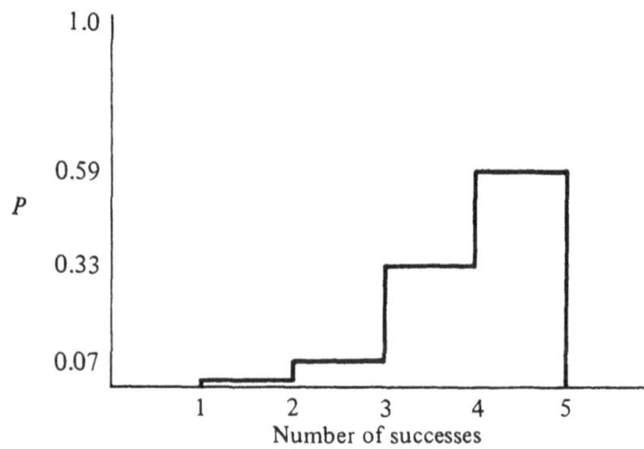

This is called a discrete distribution because there are only two possible outcomes to each trial: either the missile works, or it doesn't.

PROBLEMS

1. In the preceding example, if the reliability is 0.9, what is the probability that no more than 4 missiles will work?

   a. 0.590.
   b. 0.410.
   c. 0.672.
   d. 0.328.
   e. 0.409.

2. In which of the following measurements would the binomial distribution be appropriate?

a. Temperature fluctuations.
b. Miles per gallon of an automobile.
c. Distance between two points.
d. None of the above.
e. All of the above.

Check your answers.

Answers

1. b.

$$P(\text{no more than } 4) = 1 - P(\text{exactly } 5).$$

2. d.
None of the answers given represent discrete variables, even though discrete numbers are used to represent them. The interval between 70°F and 71°F, for example, can be subdivided infinitely.

F. NORMAL DISTRIBUTION

A common continuous distribution is the normal distribution.

> The *normal distribution* is used for continuously varying measurements.

Example

Suppose a manufacturer of micrometers wishes to check their accuracy by measuring a job block with a known thickness of 0.500 inches. Ten micrometers yield the following data:

micrometer	*reading*	*micrometer*	*reading*
1	0.501	6	0.502
2	0.498	7	0.500
3	0.499	8	0.501
4	0.500	9	0.499
5	0.500	10	0.500

A histogram of the above data looks like this:

```
              X
              X
        X     X     X
  X     X     X     X     X
-----------------------------
0.498 0.499 0.500 0.501 0.502
```

The *median* of these data is 0.500. There are as many data points above the median as there are below it.

The *mean* of the data is also 0.500. The mean is the arithmetic average of all of the datum points.

The *mode* of the data is also 0.500. The mode is the point where the greatest number of datum points are observed.

The *range* of this data is 0.004, the difference between the highest and lowest reading. The lowest reading plus half the range equals the median.

These relationships between median, mean, mode, and range are peculiar to the normal distribution. Other continuous distributions are called skewed distributions.

If we enclose the histogram with a symmetrical bell-shaped curve, we have what is called the normal distribution:

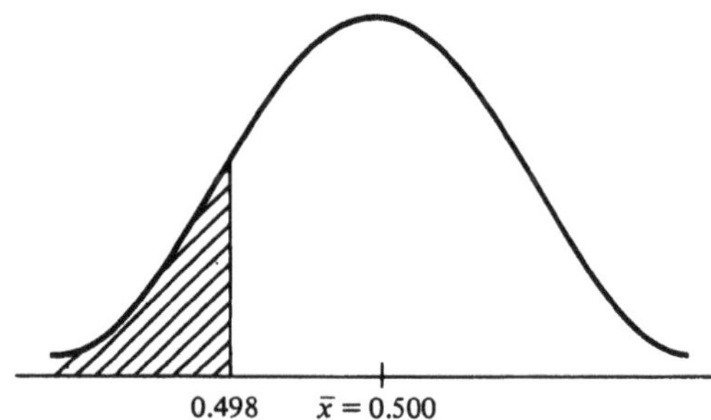

Here, $\bar{x}$ is the mean or arithmetic average of the data. The shaded area on the left represents the probability of getting a reading less than or equal to 0.498. This can be estimated numerically by calculating the variance or the standard deviation (a measure of dispersion or spread of the distribution).

$$\text{Var} = \sigma^2.$$

$$\sigma = \sqrt{\frac{\sum_{i=1}^{n} (x_i - \bar{x})^2}{n}}$$

In the example above,

$$\sum_{i=1}^{n} (x_i - \bar{x})^2 = 4(0.001)^2 + 2(0.002)^2$$

$$= 4 \times 10^{-6} + 8 \times 10^{-6}$$

$$= 12 \times 10^{-6}$$

$$\sigma = \sqrt{\frac{12 \times 10^{-6}}{10}} = 0.00109.$$

With the normal distribution, the probability of a reading within the given limits is as shown below:

$$\bar{x} \pm \sigma \qquad P = 0.6826$$

$$\bar{x} \pm 2\sigma \qquad P = 0.9544$$

$$\bar{x} \pm 3\sigma \qquad P = 0.9974.$$

PROBLEMS

1. In the skewed distribution shown below, which of the following statements is correct?

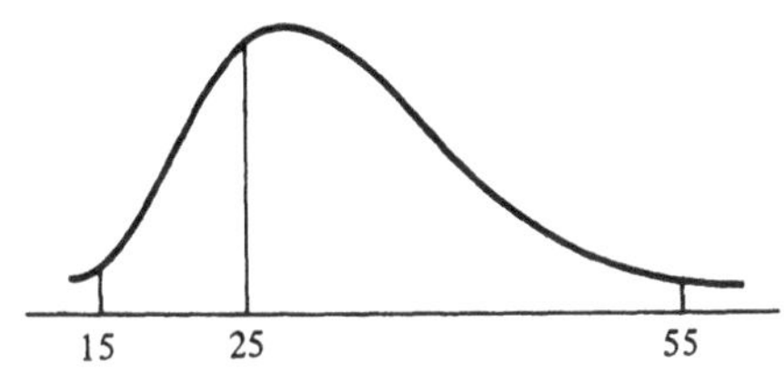

   a. The median is higher than the mean.
   b. $\bar{x}$ is greater than 25.
   c. The range is 40.
   d. $\bar{x} + \sigma$ contains 84% of the data.
   e. The mode is 35.

2. In a normal distribution, $\bar{x} = 100$ and $\sigma = 10$. Out of 1,000 observations, how many would you expect to find greater than 120?

   a. 13.
   b. 36.
   c. 114.
   d. 23.
   e. 95.

Check your answers.

Answers

1. b.
2. d.

3 Trigonometry

Discussion of and problems related to the Pythagorean Theorem; sine and cosine; tangent, cotangent, secant, and cosecant; complementary angles; radians; inverse trigonometric functions; laws of sines and cosines; and the rule of similar triangles.

Trigonometry allows us to write a functional relationship, i.e., an algebraic expression about the parameters of a triangle.

A. PYTHAGOREAN THEOREM

About 500 B.C. Pythagoras discovered the relationship between the sides of a right triangle, i.e., a triangle which has one 90° angle. In the triangle below, x and y represent the sides adjacent to the right angle and r represents the hypotenuse:

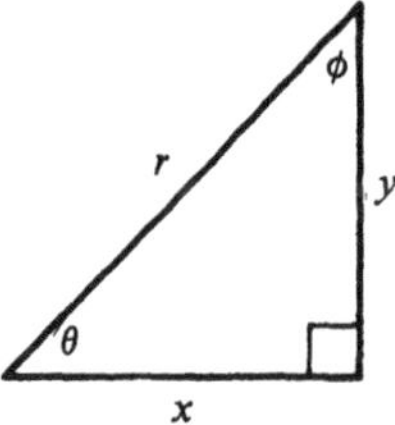

> The *Pythagorean Theorem* states:
>
> $$x^2 + y^2 = r^2.$$

Example

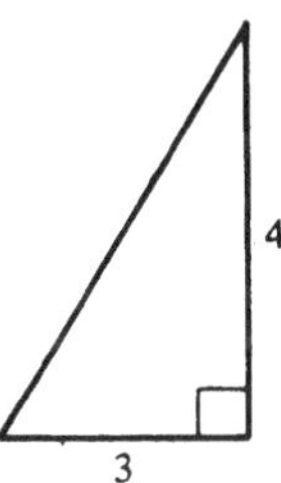

The hypotenuse is $r = \sqrt{3^2 + 4^2} = 5$.

PROBLEMS

1. The side x in triangle B below is

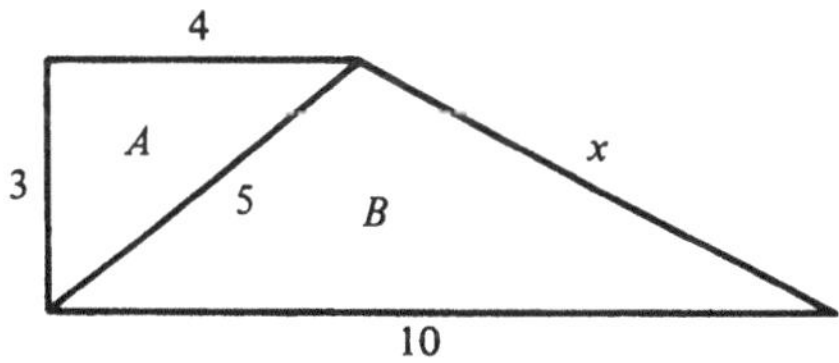

a. $\sqrt{125}$.
b. $5\sqrt{5}$.
c. $3\sqrt{5/3}$.
d. $15/\sqrt{5}$.
e. $5\sqrt{3}$.

2. A triangular plot of land contains 7000 square yards and has a hypotenuse of 172 yards. Its other two sides are nearest to:

a. 90 yds and 155 yds.
b. 100 yds and 140 yds.
c. 120 yds and 120 yds.
d. 140 yds and 170 yds.
e. 80 yds and 175 yds.

Check your answers.

Answers

1. d.
Triangle B is not a right triangle, so the Pythagorean Theorem does not apply, but one can construct a right triangle and apply the Pythagorean Theorem to it:

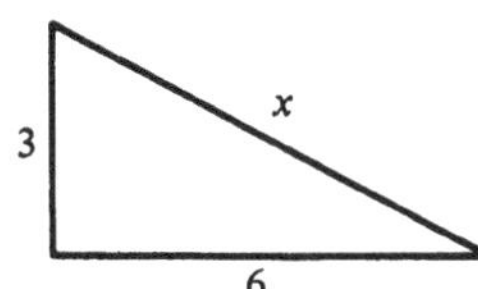

This is one method of operating on oblique triangles.

2. b.
   Area of triangle $\frac{1}{2}bh = 7000$. This is one equation in two unknowns. The Pythagorean Theorem provides another equation in the same two unknowns:

$$b^2 + h^2 = (172)^2.$$

   Solve these two simultaneously.
   If you had difficulty with this problem, review p. 10.

B. SINE AND COSINE

The Pythagorean Theorem is limited to operations involving only the sides of a triangle. The main tool of trigonometry is a transcendental function which relates the angles of a triangle to the sides. In other words, based on the triangle shown below

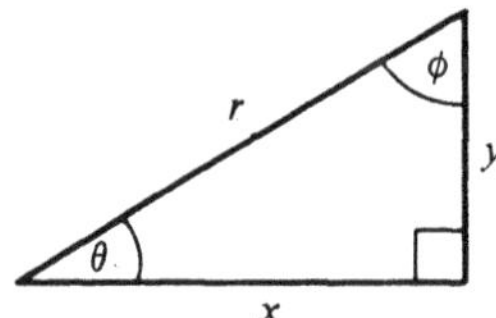

define a transcendental function in the form

$$\theta = f(x,y,r)$$

and

$$\phi = f(x,y,r).$$

This is done on the basis of a unit circle containing the above triangle:

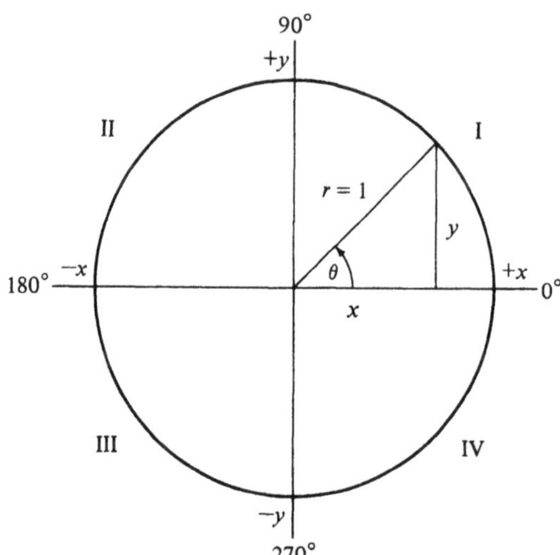

Based on this triangle, the two basic trigonometric functions are defined as follows:

$$\sin\theta = \frac{y}{r} = y$$

$$\cos\theta = \frac{x}{r} = x$$

where $\sin\theta$ is called the *sine* of θ and $\cos\theta$ is called the *cosine* of θ.

Example

What is the graphical representation of the sine and cosine between $\theta = 0°$ and $\theta = 360°$?

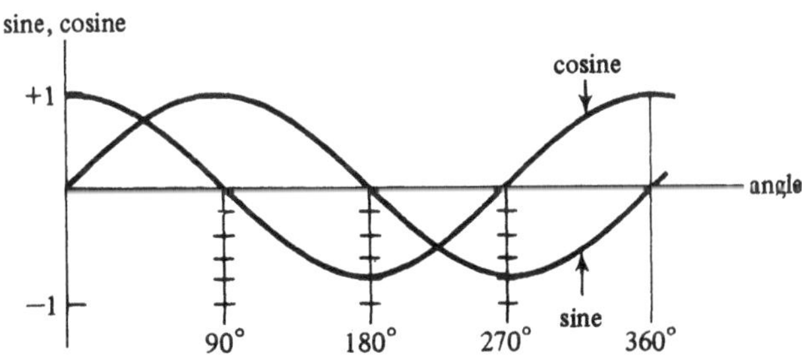

Note that the sine and cosine both vary between 1 and −1 and that they are 90° apart on the abscissa.

PROBLEMS

1. Which of the following angles has a positive sine and a negative cosine?

   a. 120°.
   b. 90°.
   c. 285°.
   d. 30°.
   e. 340°.

2. The sine of 20° is 0.342; what is the cosine of 20°?

   a. 0.658.
   b. 0.707.
   c. 0.940.
   d. 0.866.
   e. 0.174.

3. Given cosine 40° = 0.766, which angles have a sine of 0.766?

   a. 220°.
   b. 130°, 50°.
   c. 13°, 103°.
   d. 130°.
   e. None of the above.

Check your answers.

Answers

1. a.
   You can answer this by examining the graph or by using the unit circle which is the basic definition of either the sine or the cosine.
2. c.
   Based on the basic definitions, you have a triangle as shown below.

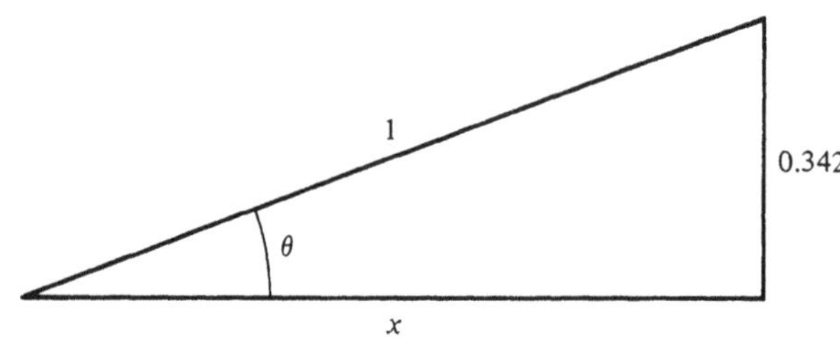

$$\cos\theta = x = \sqrt{1^2 - (0.342)^2} = 0.940.$$

3. b.
   The cosine curve is 90° ahead of the sine curve; this results in relationships such as

$$\cos\theta = \sin(90^\circ + \theta)$$
$$\sin\theta = \cos(90^\circ - \theta).$$

   You may wish to refer to a trigonometry text for a complete list of these reduction formulas.

C. TANGENT, COTANGENT, SECANT, COSECANT

The two basic trigonometric functions are the sine and the cosine. Another set of nomenclature defining them is on the basis of the following right triangle:

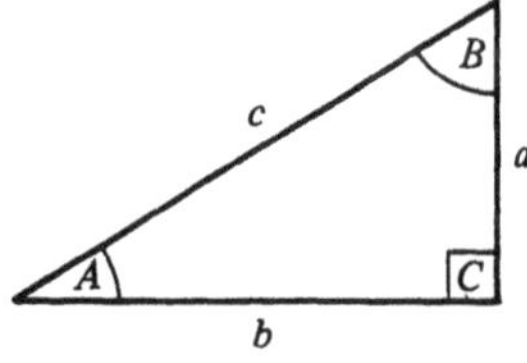

where a capital letter denotes an angle and the corresponding lower-case letter denotes the side opposite that angle. In addition to the sine and cosine, four other trigonometric functions can be defined.

$$\text{Sine } A = \sin A = \frac{a}{c} = \frac{\text{side opposite } A}{\text{hypotenuse}}$$

$$\text{Cosine } A = \cos A = \frac{b}{c} = \frac{\text{side adjacent } A}{\text{hypotenuse}}$$

$$\text{Tangent } A = \tan A = \frac{a}{b} = \frac{\sin A}{\cos A}$$

$$\text{Cotangent } A = \cot A = \frac{b}{a} = \frac{1}{\tan A}$$

$$\text{Secant } A = \sec A = \frac{c}{b} = \frac{1}{\cos A}$$

$$\text{Cosecant } A = \csc A = \frac{c}{a} = \frac{1}{\sin A}$$

Use a set of trigonometric tables or a calculator to determine the values of these functions for angles between 0° and 90°. Use the reduction formulas to determine the trigonometric functions for angles greater than 90°.

Example

Use the unit circle of p. 28 to plot the $\tan \theta$ as a function of θ.

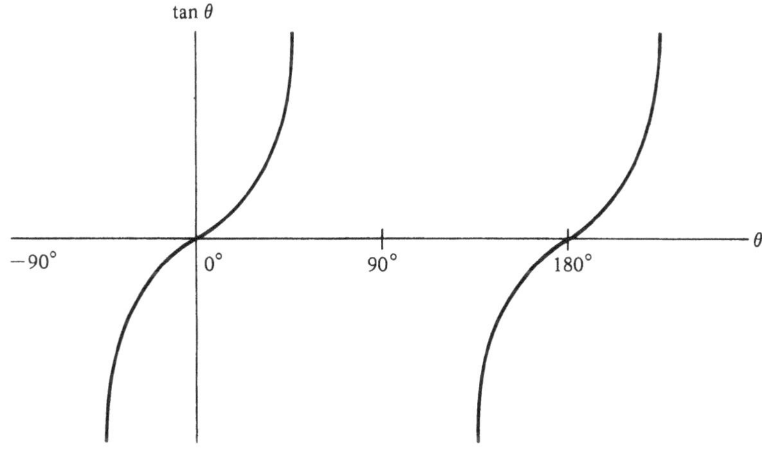

Note that the $\tan \theta \longrightarrow \pm\infty$ when $\theta \longrightarrow \pm 90°$. This is because the side adjacent to θ approaches 0.

PROBLEMS

1. All trigonometric functions:

   a. Are directly proportional to the corresponding angle.
   b. Repeat themselves every 180°.
   c. Are a ratio of linear distances.

d. Can have any positive or negative value.
e. Can equal zero.

2. $\sec^2 \theta$ equals:

a. $1 + \tan^2 \theta$.
b. $1/\csc^2 \theta$.
c. $\sin^2 \theta + \cos^2 \theta$.
d. ∞.
e. $1/\sin^2 \theta$.

Check your answers.

Answers

1. c.
The other answers are wrong because:
a. trigonometric functions are proportional to sides, not angles;
b. sines and cosines repeat every 360°;
d. sines and cosines are always one or less;
e. secants and cosecants never equal zero.
2. a.
Pythagorean Theorem $a^2 + b^2 = c^2$;
$\div$ by c^2:

$$\sin^2 \theta + \cos^2 \theta = 1;$$

$\div$ by $\cos^2 \theta$:

$$\tan^2 \theta + 1 = \frac{1}{\cos^2 \theta} = \sec^2 \theta.$$

D. COMPLEMENTARY ANGLES

In the previous sections it was established that the sine and cosine were 90° apart, leading to reduction formulas. This is also established by the definitions based on the ABC triangle, since

$$\sin B = \frac{b}{c} = \cos A.$$

In such a case A and B are said to be complementary angles. By definition the sum of all angles in any triangle equals 180°. In a right triangle, angle C equals 90°. Therefore,

A and B are complementary if $A + B = 90°$.

Example

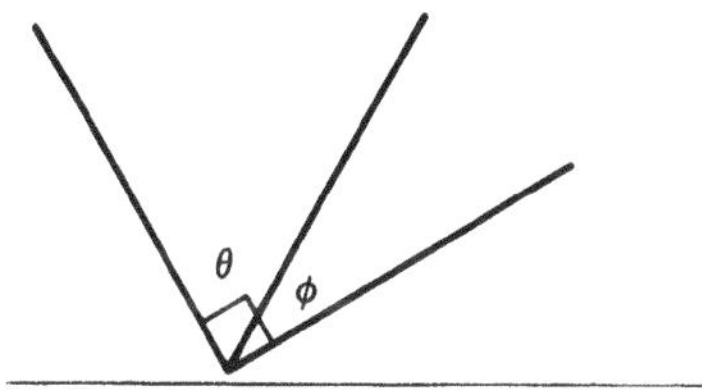

if $\theta = 60$ then $\phi = 30°$ and $\sin 60° = \cos 30°$.

PROBLEMS

1. In the figure below, solve for d.

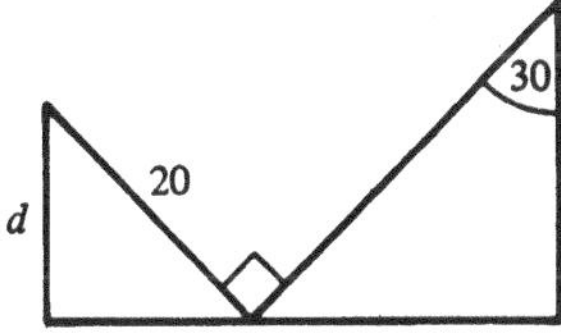

   a. 20 cos 60.
   b. sin 60/20.
   c. 20 cos 30.
   d. All of the above.
   e. None of the above.

2. The altitude of an equilateral unit triangle is:

   a. $3/\sqrt{2}$.
   b. $1/\sqrt{3}$.
   c. $\sqrt{3}/2$.
   d. $\sqrt{2}/3$.
   e. $1/\sqrt{2}$.

Check your answers.

Answers

1. a.
   By complementary angles, the triangle is:

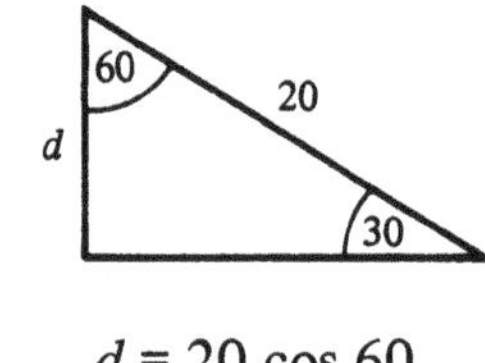

$$d = 20 \cos 60.$$

2. c.

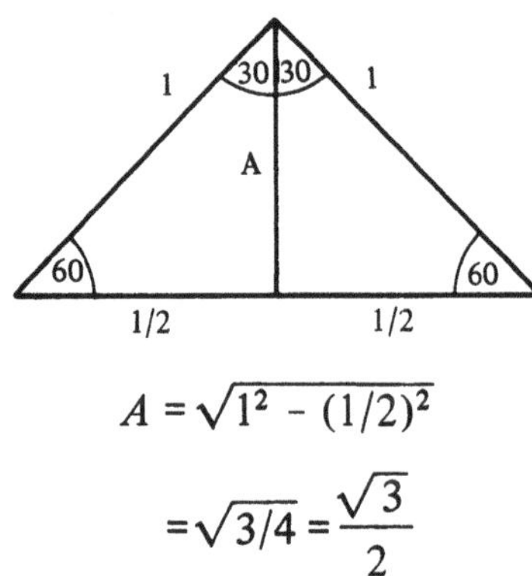

$$A = \sqrt{1^2 - (1/2)^2}$$

$$= \sqrt{3/4} = \frac{\sqrt{3}}{2}$$

E. RADIANS

The common measure of angles is the degree. The angular degree is $\frac{1}{360}$ of a full circle. (The degree has its origin in the duodecimal numbering system of the ancient Sumerians.)

The circular mil is also sometimes used to measure angles. A circular mil equals $\frac{1}{6400}$ of the circumference of a circle.

Both the angular degree and the circular mil represent a unit or dimension. The radian, however, is a dimensionless and much more basic angular measure. The radian of an angle subtending an arc s is defined as follows:

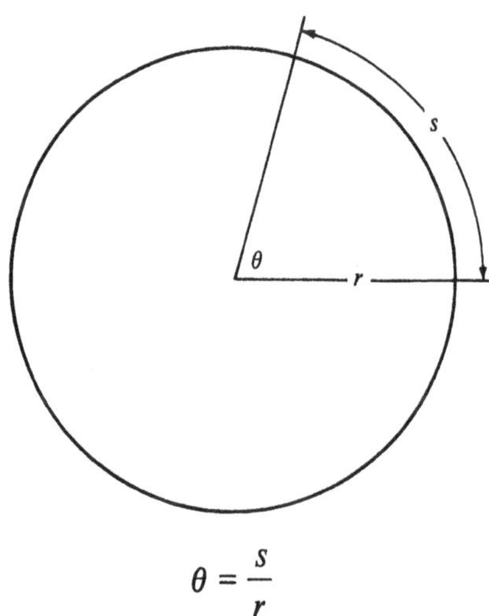

$$\theta = \frac{s}{r}$$

θ is dimensionless because it is the ratio of two linear measurements. This attribute is important in working certain engineering formulas because one does not have to deal with the angular measurement as a unit but can use it as a pure dimensionless number. Since angles are not commonly measured in radians, a conversion must usually be made. The conversion is based on the circumference of a circle ($2\pi r$).

$$\boxed{360^\circ = 2\pi \text{ radians.}}$$

Example

Convert 60° into radians.

$$(60^\circ)\ \frac{2\pi \text{ radians}}{360^\circ} = 1.05 \text{ radians.}$$

PROBLEMS

1. What is the rotational velocity in radians per second of a wheel rotating at 1800 rpm?

   a. 10,805 per sec.
   b. 30 per sec.
   c. 67,858 per sec.
   d. 377 per sec.
   e. 188 per sec.

2. The sine of 1.75π is:

   a. 0.707.
   b. -1.414.
   c. 0.500.
   d. -0.707.
   e. 0.867.

Check your answers.

Answers

1. e.
2. d.

   If you had difficulty with these problems, review p. 34.

F. INVERSE TRIGONOMETRIC FUNCTIONS

An expression involving a trigonometric function is usually written as

$$\sin 30^\circ = \tfrac{1}{2}.$$

Writing the same expression using the inverse trigonometric function results in:

$$\boxed{\text{Arc sine } \tfrac{1}{2} = \sin^{-1} \tfrac{1}{2} = 30°.}$$

Example

$$\tan^{-1} 1.732 = 60$$

PROBLEMS

1. $\tan(\sin^{-1} 0.966 - \cos^{-1} 0.500)$ equals:

   a. 60°.
   b. 0.268.
   c. 45°.
   d. 0.866.
   e. ∞.

2. If $\csc \phi = \sqrt{(x^2 + y^2)}/y$, then:

   a. $\cot^{-1} \dfrac{x}{y} = \dfrac{\pi}{2} - \phi.$
   b. $\tan^{-1} \dfrac{x}{y} = \phi.$
   c. $\sin^{-1} \dfrac{x}{\sqrt{x^2 + y^2}} = \pi/2 - \phi.$
   d. None of the above.
   e. All of the above.

Check your answers.

Answers

1. b.
   Refer to pp. 30–31.
2. c.
   Refer to p. 31.

G. LAWS OF SINES AND COSINES

All trigonometric functions are defined on the basis of a right triangle and therefore can only be applied directly to solutions of right triangles. A right triangle is unique in that one of its angles has a known magnitude, 90°. To solve a right triangle, you need to know only two additional quantities–two sides, or one side and an angle.

To solve an oblique triangle, you must know one additional quantity because the three angles can have any value. Oblique triangles are solved by using either the *Law of Sines* or the *Law of Cosines.* Based on the oblique *ABC* triangle below,

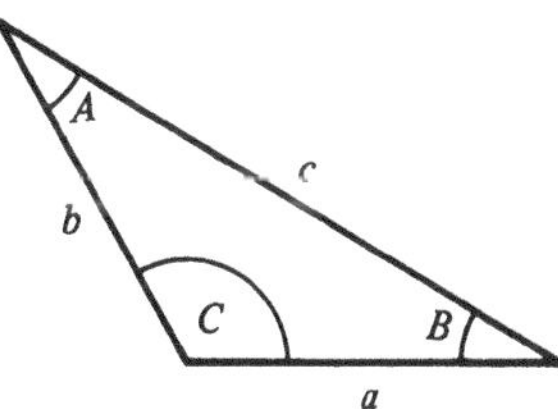

Law of Sines:

$$\frac{\sin A}{a} = \frac{\sin B}{b} = \frac{\sin C}{c}$$

Law of Cosines:

$$a^2 = b^2 + c^2 - 2bc \cos A$$

Example

Generalize the Law of Cosines to cover the case where angle B and sides a and c are known.

The result is

$$b^2 = c^2 + a^2 - 2ca \cos B.$$

PROBLEMS

1.

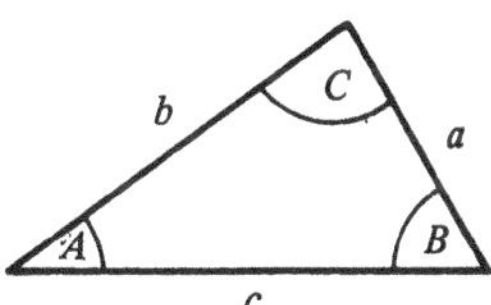

In the triangle above, angle A, side b, and side a are known. Which of the following expressions are true for side c?

a. $c^2 = b^2 + a^2 - 2ba \cos A$.

b. $c = \dfrac{(\sin A)(b)}{(a)}$.

c. $c^2 = a^2 + b^2 - 2ac \cos A$.

d. All of the above.

e. None of the above.

2.

Find the distance across the river from A to B.

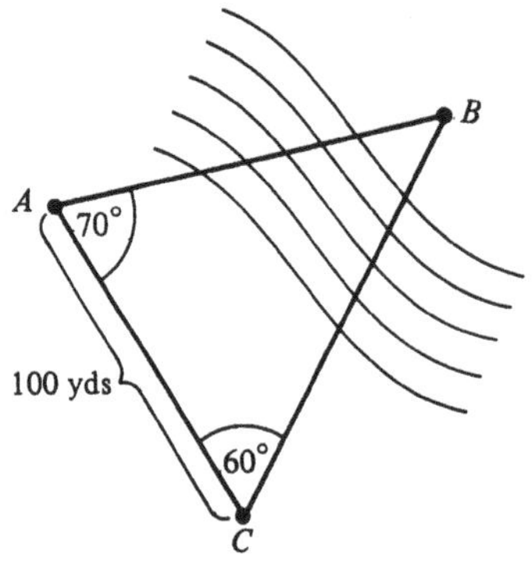

a. 113 yds.
b. 108 yds.
c. 92 yds.
d. 88 yds.
e. 122 yds.

Check your answers.

Answers

1. e.
Solve for side c as a function of angle C using the Law of Sines:

$$C = \frac{(\text{Sine } C)(a)}{(\text{Sine } A)}, \qquad \text{where sin } A \text{ is unknown.}$$

Solve simultaneously with

$$a^2 = b^2 + c^2 - 2bc \cos A.$$

2. a.
First determine the value of the third angle; then apply the Law of Sines.

H. RULE OF SIMILAR TRIANGLES

A powerful tool for solving both oblique and right triangles is the *Rule of Similar Triangles.* Two triangles are similar if their angles are equal. If two triangles are similar, their sides are proportional. In the two triangles below,

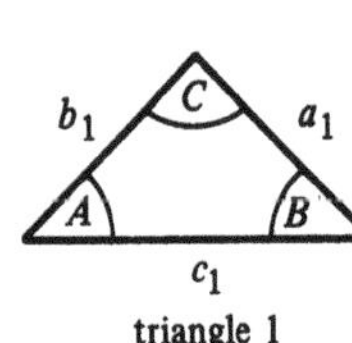

triangle 1

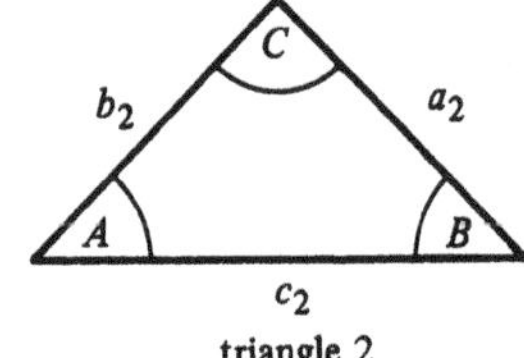

triangle 2

$$\frac{a_1}{a_2} = \frac{b_1}{b_2} = \frac{c_1}{c_2}.$$

Example

The distance d in the situation below is:

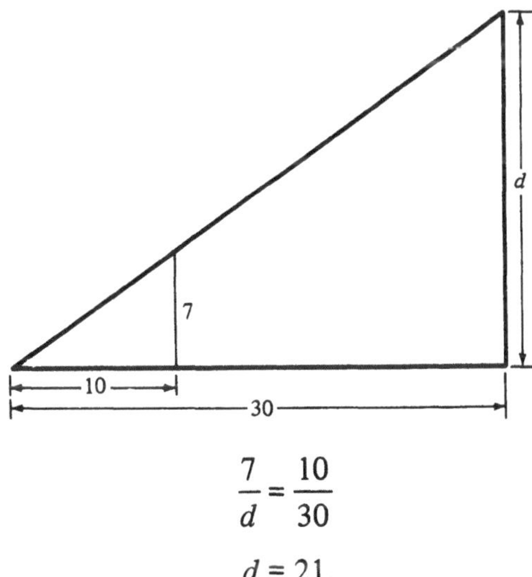

$$\frac{7}{d} = \frac{10}{30}$$

$$d = 21.$$

PROBLEM

1. The distance d in the figure below is nearest to:

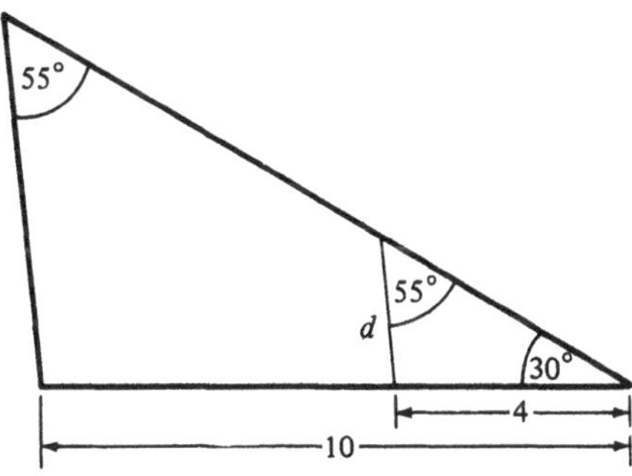

a. 3.
b. 5.
c. 6.
d. 4.
e. 2.

Check your answer.

Answer

1. e.

$$d = 2.4415 \text{ exactly}.$$

4 Analytic Geometry

Discussion of and problems related to the distance between two points, loci, equation of a straight line, slope of a straight line, the circle, and other second-degree polynomials.

A. DEFINITION

Analytic geometry is an extension of trigonometry; while trigonometry deals with straight lines and angles, analytic geometry deals with all geometric figures. The Greeks of Euclid's time studied the properties of geometric figures, but, lacking algebra, they were forced to use nonquantitative techniques, i.e., Euclidian geometry, sometimes called plane geometry. In the 17th Century Descartes developed a study of geometry using the tools of algebra, i.e., analytic geometry.

Descartes' basic tool is the Cartesian coordinate system which is basically a map of two-dimensional space upon which geometric figures can be located. The location of the simplest figure, a point, is defined by its x and y coordinates. For instance, the point defined by the intersection of lines $x = 3$ and $y = 5$ has coordinates 3 and 5. This is written as $P_{(3,5)}$. Graphically in Cartesian space it is shown as follows:

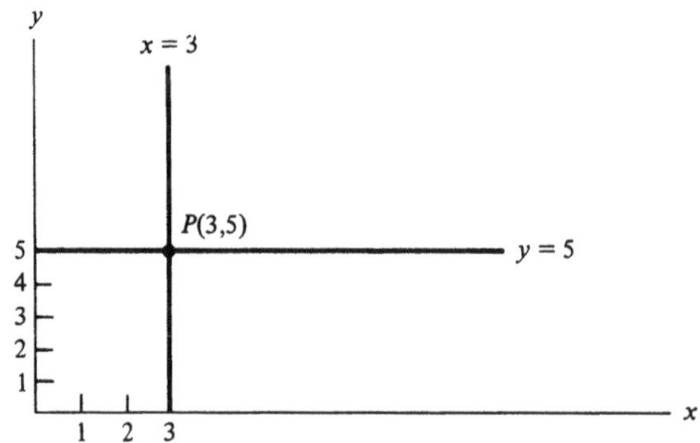

$P_{(x,y)}$ represents a point with coordinates x and y.

Example

Point 1 which is at an unknown location would be written as

$$P(x_1, y_1)$$

and represents the intersection of lines

$$x = x_1$$

and

$$y = y_1.$$

PROBLEM

A ship is heading due NE from a position $P(5,50)$. When its longitude is 10°E its latitude is:

a. 45°N.
b. 55°N.
c. 48°N.
d. 45°S.
e. The ship is on a mountain top in Sweden.

Check your answer.

Answer

b.
You may want to refer to basic geographical coordinate definitions to help relate them to the Cartesian coordinate system. The equator is equivalent to the x axis, and a North–South line through Greenwich, England, is equivalent to the y axis.

B. DISTANCE BETWEEN TWO POINTS

If the locations of two points are known, the next logical question concerns the distance between them. In the figure below the distance between P_1 and P_2 is found by the Pythagorean Theorem.

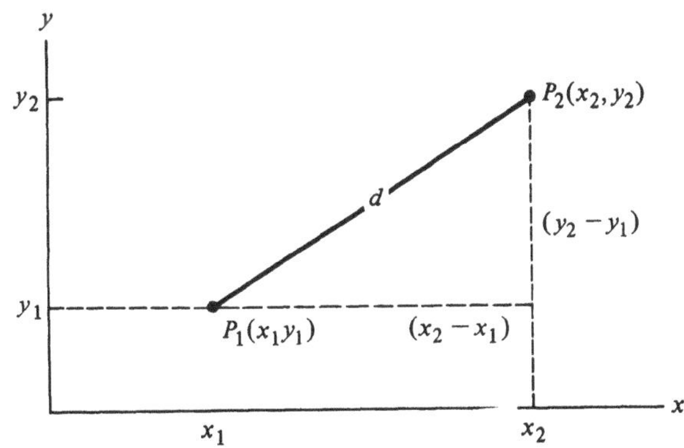

Distance:

$$d = \sqrt{(x_2 - x_1)^2 + (y_2 - y_1)^2}$$

Example

If P_1 has coordinates (3,2) and P_2 has coordinates (5,3), then

$$d = \sqrt{(5-3)^2 + (3-2)^2}$$

$$= \sqrt{2^2 + 1^2}$$

$$= \sqrt{5}.$$

PROBLEM

The distance between $P(2,3)$ and $P(-1,2)$ is:

a. 1.41.
b. 2.83.
c. 4.89.
d. 4.00.
e. 3.16.

Check your answer.

Answer

e.
If you had trouble with this problem, you probably (a) were not consistent in defining point 1 and point 2, OR (b) made an error in the sign of a number during manipulation.

C. LOCI

The Latin word *locus* is the root of the English word *location.* A moving point has a location in Cartesian coordinates at any point in time. If these locations were plotted, the result would be a line; therefore, a locus is a line in space.

A *locus* is a path made by a point moving in accordance with a rule.

Example

Find the locus of a point (P) which moves so that it is always equidistant from two fixed points, $A_{(1,2)}$ and $B_{(-1,0)}$.

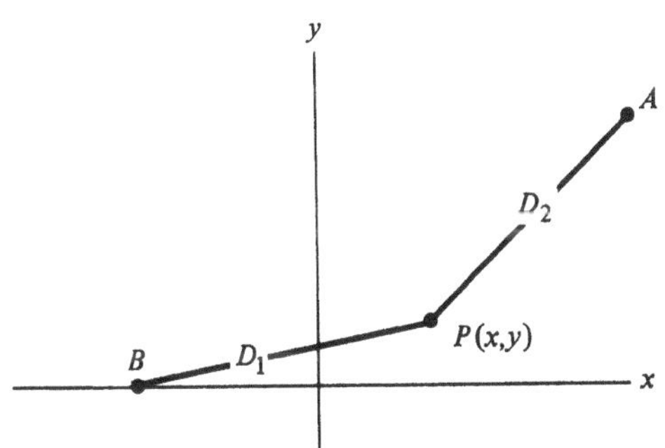

From the statement we know that D_1 always equals D_2:

$$D_1 = D_2 \quad \text{or} \quad \sqrt{(x-1)^2 + (y-2)^2} = \sqrt{(x+1)^2 + y^2}\,.$$

Reducing this results in the following:

$$x^2 - 2x + 1 + y^2 - 4y + 4 = x^2 + 2x + 1 + y^2$$

or

$$x + y - 1 = 0$$

the equation of a straight line.

PROBLEMS

1. What is the locus of a point which is always equidistant from the point $P(1,1)$ and the line $x = 0$?

   a. Circle.
   b. Ellipse.
   c. Straight line.
   d. Parabola.
   e. Involute.

2. What is the nearest circumference of a circle generated by a point always 3 units from $P(5,5)$?

   a. 19.
   b. 8.
   c. 9.
   d. 16.
   e. None of the above.

Check your answers.

Answers

1. d.
   This locus can be determined graphically, or you could refer to an analytic geometry text. The eccentricity of a figure is defined as the ratio of the distance from a point to the distance from a line. A parabola is the only figure with an eccentricity of 1.
2. a.
   The distance from the fixed point to the moving point is the *radius* of the circle.

D. EQUATION OF A STRAIGHT LINE

A linear algebraic equation in two unknowns forms a straight line if plotted in the Cartesian coordinate system.

The equation $x + y = 3$ plots as:

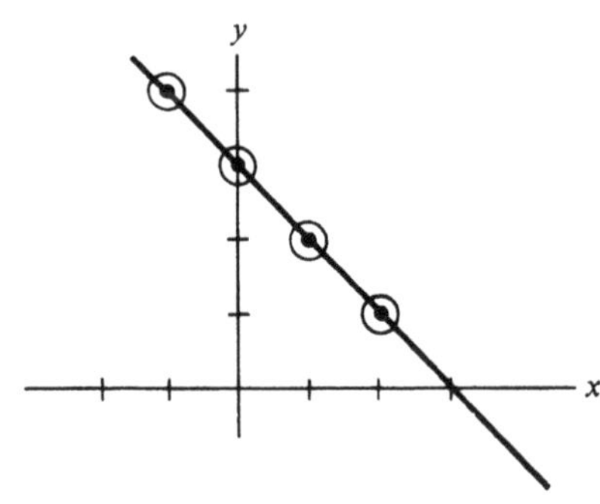

> The equation for a straight line is in the form
>
> $$Ax + By + C = 0,$$
>
> where A, B, and C are constant coefficients.

Example

The form of the equation for a straight line is $Ax + By + C = 0$. If the line is defined by the two points $P_1 = (2,1)$ and $P_2 = (-6,5)$ (see below)

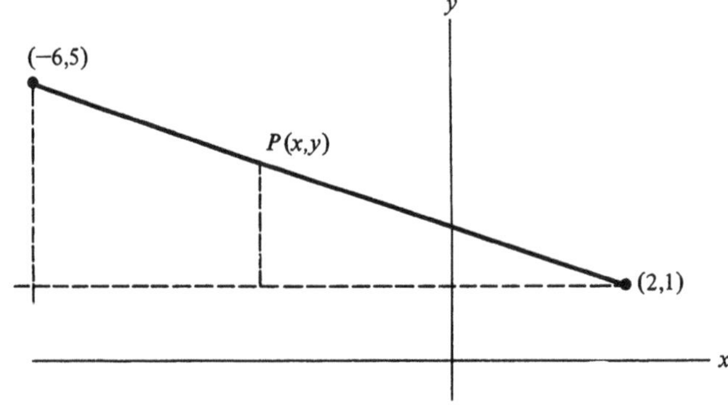

then, by similar triangles,

$$\frac{y - 1}{x - 2} = \frac{5 - 1}{-6 - 2},$$

which reduces to $x + 2y - 4 = 0$.

PROBLEMS

1. A line intersects the curve $y = x^2 - 2$ at point $P(3,y)$ and also passes through point $P(1,0)$. Its equation is:

   a. $y - 3x + 14 = 0$.
   b. $7y - 3x + 21 = 0$.
   c. $2y - 7x + 7 = 0$.
   d. $y - 3x + 21 = 0$.
   e. $2y - 7x - 14 = 0$.

2. Which of the following equations represents a straight line?

   a. $x = \sqrt{y - 3}$.
   b. $\sqrt{x^2 + 4} = y$.
   c. $\sqrt{x + 4} = \sqrt{y - 3}$.
   d. All of the above.
   e. None of the above.

Check your answers.

Answers

1. c.
   Use the two-point method described in the example. One point is determined by the simultaneous solution of $y = x^2 - 2$ and $x = 3$.
2. c.
   If both sides are squared, you have $x - y + 7 = 0$.

E. SLOPE OF A STRAIGHT LINE

The slope of a line is defined as the tangent of the angle of inclination to the x axis.

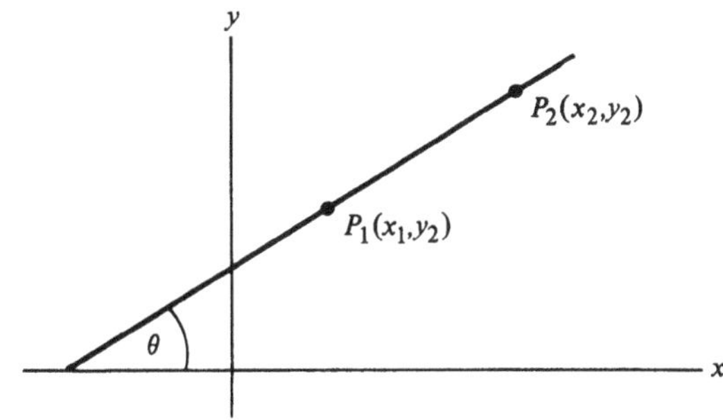

Slope:

$$m = \tan \theta$$
$$= \frac{y_2 - y_1}{x_2 - x_1} = \frac{\Delta y}{\Delta x}$$

The slope of a line is a component in another standard form of the equation of a straight line:

$$y = mx + b,$$
where m is the slope and b is the y intercept.

Example

A straight line is defined by a slope and one point:

$$P = (3,-4)$$
$$\text{slope} = \frac{\Delta y}{\Delta x} = \sqrt{3} \qquad (\theta = 60^\circ).$$

Its equation is derived as follows:

$$\frac{\Delta y}{\Delta x} = \sqrt{3} = \frac{y + 4}{x - 3}$$
$$y = \sqrt{3}x - 3\sqrt{3} - 4.$$

PROBLEMS

1. If a line has slope m, the slope of a line normal to it is:

   a. $-m$.
   b. $-1/m$.
   c. $1/m$.
   d. m.
   e. b/m.

2. The normal distance from $x - y - 5 = 0$ to $P(3,4)$ is nearest to:

   a. 5.7.
   b. 8.5.
   c. 3.5.
   d. 4.8.
   e. 4.2.

Check your answers.

Answers

1. b.
   Refer to a text or dictionary for a definition of "normal"; then use the rules of complimentary angles to determine the slope.
2. e.
   Refer to problem 1 for a definition of "normal." Refer to section D for the point of intersection. Refer to section B for the distance.

F. THE CIRCLE

Any polynomial equation of degree 2 or higher forms a curved line when plotted in the Cartesian coordinate system. The most common example of a second degree polynomial is the circle. The locus definition of a circle is the path made by a point moving about a fixed point in such a way that they are always equidistant. The fixed point is the center of the circle; the distance is the radius of the circle. A circle is fully defined by the center and the radius.

Standard form of the equation of a circle:

$$x^2 + y^2 + ax + by + c = 0.$$

Location of the center:

$$x = -a/2$$

$$y = -b/2.$$

$$\text{Radius} = \sqrt{\frac{a^2 + b^2 - 4c}{4}}.$$

Example

Find the center and radius of the circle

$$2x^2 + 2y^2 - 5x + 4y - 7 = 0.$$

Normalizing,

$$x^2 + y^2 - \frac{5}{2}x + 2y = \frac{7}{2}$$

or

$$a = -\frac{5}{2}, \quad b = 2, \quad c = -\frac{7}{2}.$$

The center then is

$$x = \frac{5}{4}$$

$$y = -1$$

and

$$r = \sqrt{\frac{\left(-\frac{5}{2}\right)^2 + (2)^2 + \frac{(4)(7)}{2}}{4}}$$

$$= \sqrt{\frac{97}{16}} = \frac{1}{4}\sqrt{97}.$$

PROBLEMS

1. Which of the following points are the center of a circle through $P(-1,2)$ and tangent to the axes?

   a. (-1,1).
   b. (-5,1).
   c. (-1,5).
   d. (0,1).
   e. (-5,0).

2. Find a point of tangency between $x^2 + y^2 - 3x + 2 = 0$ and $2y - x + 2 = 0$.

   a. (-2,0).
   b. (1,1).
   c. (3,-2).
   d. (2,0).
   e. None of the above.

Check your answers.

Answers

1. a.
   Start by defining the radius as the distance from the point to the center. Then equate that expression with the distance to either axes.
2. d.
   The points of tangency are the simultaneous solution of these two polynomials.

G. OTHER SECOND-DEGREE POLYNOMIALS

The circle is the only second-degree polynomial which is symmetrical about any line drawn through its centroid. Three other common second-degree polynomials which do not have this property are the parabola, the ellipse, and the hyperbola. The equations for these figures when their main axis of symmetry is parallel to the x axis are presented below. Note how they differ from each other and how they differ from the equation for a circle.

Parabola:

$$(y - k)^2 = 4p(x - h).$$

Ellipse:

$$\frac{(x - h)^2}{a^2} + \frac{(y - k)^2}{b^2} = 1.$$

Hyperbola:

$$\frac{(x - h)^2}{a^2} - \frac{(y - k)^2}{b^2} = 1.$$

Example

The shape of a figure can be deduced from the form of the equation. The polynomial $x^2 + 2y^2 - 3 = 0$ forms an ellipse since the coefficients of x^2 and y^2 are unequal and of the same sign.

PROBLEMS

1. The equation $x^2 = 4y$ represents:

   a. A hyperbola parallel to the x axis.
   b. A hyperbola parallel to the y axis.
   c. A parabola parallel to the x axis.
   d. A parabola parallel to the y axis.
   e. An ellipse parallel to the x axis.

2. A three-dimensional paraboloid $x^2 + y^2 = 4z$ is cut by a plane $y = 2x$. The resulting figure is:

   a. Hyperbola.
   b. Parabola.
   c. Circle.
   d. Ellipse.
   e. Involute.

Check your answers.

Answers

1. d.
   Either deduce the answer from the equations given, or refer to a more complete text on analytic geometry.
2. b.
   Solve the two equations simultaneously and examine the form of the resulting two-dimensional equation.

5 Differential Calculus

Discussion of and problems related to the slope of a curved line, differentiation of polynomial terms, differentiation of algebraic expressions, related rates, implicit differentiation, partial differentiation, maxima and minima, differentiation of trigonometric functions, and differentials.

A. DEFINITION

Differential calculus is the study of the rate of change of one variable with respect to another. Newton is generally credited with developing differential calculus to aid in developing the Laws of Motion. In this case, motion is defined as the rate of change of position with respect to time. Graphically, a position versus time curve looks like this:

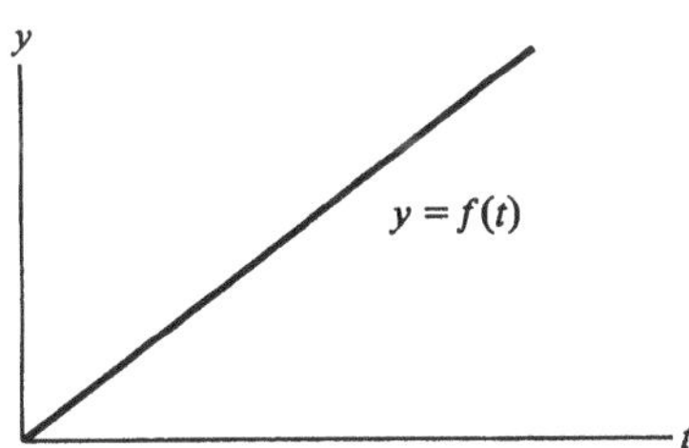

The rate of change of position y with respect to time t is represented by the slope of the line:

$$m = \frac{\Delta y}{\Delta t}.$$

Therefore, differential calculus can also be thought of as a study of slopes of lines. In the position versus time plot above, position changes linearly with time.

> In a functional relationship
>
> $$y = f(x)$$
>
> the rate of change of y with respect to x is
>
> $$\frac{\Delta y}{\Delta x} = \text{slope.}$$

Example

If $y = 2x + 1$,

$$\frac{\Delta y}{\Delta x} = 2,$$

which is the same as stating that for each unit increase in x, y increases by 2.

PROBLEM

A compression spring has a normal length of one foot and a spring constant of 3 in./lb. This could be stated algebraically as:

a. $F = 3x + 12.$
b. $F = \frac{3}{2}x^2 + 12.$
c. $F = \frac{1}{3}x.$
d. $F = 3x - 4.$
e. $F = -3x + 12.$

Check your answer.

Answer

a.
Fit this situation into the form $F = mx + b$, where m is related to the spring constant and b is the F intercept ($x = 0$).

B. SLOPE OF A CURVED LINE

The previous simple definition of slope is based on a straight line, which is unique in that its slope is the same anywhere along the line. This is *not* true for a curved line. In the case of a curved line, the slope of the line at any point along the line is equal to the slope of a line tangent to the curve at that point. Constructing tangent lines is more difficult than calculating $\Delta y/\Delta x$: if we apply the $\Delta y/\Delta x$ technique to a curved line, we do not get a true representation of slope at a point. Consider this illustration:

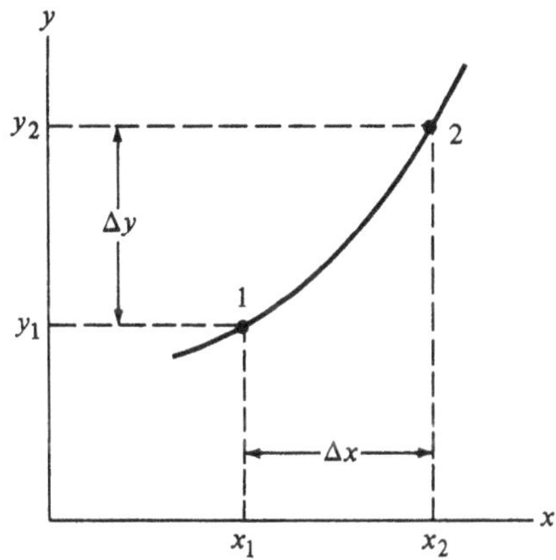

Note that the slope is steeper at (x_2,y_2) than it is at (x_1,y_1). However, this difference decreases as Δx decreases. In fact, if we move x_2 so close to x_1 that Δx approaches 0, then $\Delta y/\Delta x$ describes the slope at point 1. In other words, the slope at point 1 can be defined as the limit of $\Delta y/\Delta x$ as Δx approaches 0.

The preceding statement is the basic definition of the derivative of a function. Stated symbolically:

> In the case where $y = f(x)$, the derivative of y with respect to x is defined as:
>
> $$\frac{dy}{dx} = \lim_{\Delta x \to 0} \frac{\Delta y}{\Delta x}.$$

dy/dx is completely analogous to $\Delta y/\Delta x$ and is the slope of a curved line at a point.

The limit operation required by this definition involves determining an expression for $\Delta y/\Delta x$ and substituting $\Delta x = 0$ in the expression. This must be done carefully to avoid dividing by 0.

Example

Consider the relationship

$$y = x^2 + 2x + 3.$$

Find dy/dx at the point where $x = 1$ (point P).

Define point P as (x,y). There is also a point Q on the curve which can be defined as $(x + \Delta x), (y + \Delta y)$; graphically:

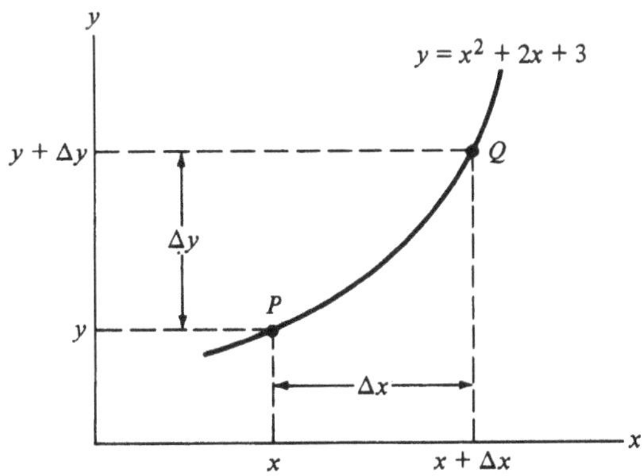

Since both points lie on the curve, we can substitute $x + \Delta x$ for x and $y + \Delta y$ for y in the equation. The equation then becomes:

$$y + \Delta y = (x + \Delta x)^2 + 2(x + \Delta x) + 3$$
$$= x^2 + 2x\Delta x + (\Delta x)^2 + 2x + 2\Delta x + 3.$$

This is an expression for $y + \Delta y$. If we subtract y from the expression, we have an expression for Δy alone. Since $y = x^2 + 2x + 3$,

$$\Delta y = 2x\Delta x + (\Delta x)^2 + 2\Delta x.$$

If we divide by Δx, we have an expression for $\Delta y/\Delta x$:

$$\frac{\Delta y}{\Delta x} = 2x + \Delta x + 2.$$

Then

$$\frac{dy}{dx} = \lim_{\Delta x \to 0} 2x + \Delta x + 2 = 2x + 2.$$

At the point $x = 1$,

$$\frac{dy}{dx} = 4.$$

PROBLEMS

1. Evaluate

$$\lim_{\Delta x \to 2} \frac{x^2 - 4}{x - 2}.$$

a. 2.
b. 0.
c. ∞.
d. 4.
e. None of the above.

2. The derivative of the function $y = 2x^2 + 3x + 1$ is:

a. $\lim_{\Delta x \to 0} 4x + 2\Delta x + 3$.
b. $4x + 3$.
c. $dy = dx(4x + 3)$.
d. All of the above.
e. None of the above.

3. Tangents to the curve $y = x^2 + 2x + 3$ at points (1,6) and (0,3) intersect at:

a. (1/2, 4).
b. (1, 3).
c. (1/2, 2).
d. (2, 4).
e. (4, 1/2).

Check your answers.

Answers

1. d.
   Rearrange the expression to avoid dividing by 0, as was done in the example.
2. d.
   Evaluate the Limit as $\Delta x \longrightarrow 0$; then complete the limit operation.
3. a.
   Use $y = mx + b$ for the tangent lines. Evaluate $dy/dx = m$ and b for each line; then solve simultaneously. You may want to refer to chapters on trigonometry and analytic geometry if you had difficulty with this problem.

C. DIFFERENTIATION OF POLYNOMIAL TERMS

Any polynomial can be expressed as $y = f(x)$. The symbols commonly used to denote the derivative of y with respect to x are

$$\frac{dy}{dx} = f'(x) = D(x) = y' = \dot{y}.$$

(The last term, $\dot{y}$, is reserved for use with respect to t–the rate of change of y with respect to t is velocity.)

If the first derivative, $y' = f'(x)$, is also a function of x, then we can differentiate again to obtain what is known as the second derivative:

$$\frac{dy'}{dx} = \frac{d^2y}{dx^2} = f''(x) = D^2(x) = y'' = \ddot{y}$$

($\ddot{y}$ is the second derivative of y with respect to time–acceleration.)

In the example of the previous section we can generalize a differentiation formula to cover polynomials of one term. In that example:

$$y = x^2 + 2x + 3$$

and

$$\frac{dy}{dx} = 2x + 2.$$

The general rule covering this operation is as follows:

If $y = x^n$, then $\dfrac{dy}{dx} = \dfrac{d(x^n)}{dx} = nx^{n-1}$.

Example

In free fall a body's position with respect to time is governed by

$$y = \tfrac{1}{2}gt^2 = 16.1t^2.$$

The body's velocity at time t is (using the above formula)

$$v = \frac{dy}{dt} = 32.2t,$$

and its acceleration is

$$a = \frac{dv}{dt} = \frac{d^2y}{dt^2} = 32.2.$$

PROBLEMS

1. If $dy/dx = 4$, the function y represents a:

   a. Circle.
   b. Tangent.
   c. Straight line.
   d. Slope.
   e. Hyperbola.

2. The first derivative of $y = (x^2 + 1)^2$ is:

   a. $2x^2 + 1$.
   b. $4x^3 + 4x$.
   c. $x^4 + 2x^2 + 1$.
   d. $4x^3 + 2x$.
   e. $x^3 + 4x + 1$.

3. In the functional relationship, which of the statements is true at point P?

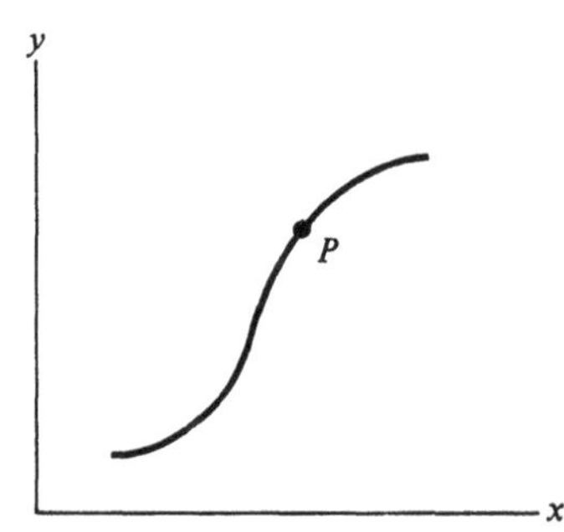

   a. y' is positive; y'' is positive.
   b. y' is negative; y'' is positive.
   c. y' is negative; y'' is negative.
   d. y' is positive; y'' is negative.
   e. y' is positive; y'' is 0.

Check your answers.

Answers

1. c.
   Refer to Section A–definition of slope for a straight line.
2. b.
   Expand the expression into a three-term polynomial; then use the general rule term by term.
3. d.
   Make a rough sketch of $y' = f'(x)$ and evaluate its slope which is y''.

D. DIFFERENTIATION OF ALGEBRAIC EXPRESSIONS

In the previous section, a formula was presented for differentiating a term in a polynomial. Using the limit theorem, formulas can be developed for other algebraic expressions. An abbreviated list of the most commonly used algebraic expressions is presented below. For a more complete listing, refer to a handbook or a calculus text.

1. $\dfrac{d}{dx}(c) = 0$, where c is any constant.

2. $\dfrac{d}{dx}(x) = 1.$

3. $\dfrac{d}{dx}(u + v + w + \cdots) = \dfrac{d}{dx}(u) + \dfrac{d}{dx}(v) + \dfrac{d}{dx}(w) + \cdots.$

4. $\dfrac{d}{dx}(cu) = c\dfrac{d(u)}{dx}.$

5. $\dfrac{d}{dx}(uv) = u\dfrac{d}{dx}(v) + v\dfrac{d}{dx}(u).$

6. $\dfrac{d}{dx}(uvw) = uv\dfrac{d}{dx}(w) + uw\dfrac{d}{dx}(v) + vw\dfrac{d}{dx}(u).$

7. $\dfrac{d}{dx}\left(\dfrac{u}{c}\right) = \dfrac{1}{c}\dfrac{d}{dx}(u).$

8. $\dfrac{d}{dx}\left(\dfrac{c}{u}\right) = c\dfrac{d}{dx}\left(\dfrac{1}{u}\right) = -\dfrac{c}{u^2}\dfrac{d(u)}{dx}.$

9. $\dfrac{d}{dx}\left(\dfrac{u}{v}\right) = \dfrac{v\dfrac{d}{dx}(u) - u\dfrac{d}{dx}(v)}{v^2}.$

10. $\dfrac{d}{dx}(x^n) = nx^{n-1}$

11. $\dfrac{d}{dx}(u^n) = nu^{n-1}\dfrac{d}{dx}(u)$

In the above formulas,

$$u = f_1(x)$$
$$v = f_2(x)$$
$$w = f_3(x).$$

Example (Using Formula 11)

$$y = (x^2 + 1)^2$$

Let $u = x^2 + 1$. Then

$$y' = 2(x^2 + 1)\frac{d(x^2 + 1)}{dx}$$

$$y' = 2(x^2 + 1)(2x)$$

Review Problem 2 in the previous section and note how the use of formula 10 differs from formula 11.

PROBLEM

Evaluate dy/dx if $y = x/\sqrt{x + 1}$.

a. $\dfrac{x\sqrt{x+1}}{(x+1)^{3/2}}$.

b. $\dfrac{\sqrt{x+1}}{x+1}$.

c. $\dfrac{x+1}{2(x+1)^{1/2}}$.

d. $\dfrac{x+2}{2(x+1)^{3/2}}$.

e. $\dfrac{x+1}{\sqrt{x+1}}$.

Check your answer.

Answer

d.
Use formula 9.

E. RELATED RATES

If two variables are related to a third variable, they can be related to each other. The manipulation required to do this depends upon being able to treat dy/dx as a fraction. This is in general permissible, and very useful. (Remember that dy/dx was derived from $\Delta y/\Delta x$, which is a fraction.)

If

$$y = f(x), \quad \frac{dy}{dx} = f'(x)$$

and

$$x = f(t), \quad \frac{dx}{dt} = f'(t)$$

then

$$\frac{dy}{dt} = \frac{dy}{dx}\,\frac{dx}{dt}.$$

Example

A point moves along the curve $y = x^3 - 3x + 5$ so that $x = \frac{1}{2}\sqrt{t} + 3$. What is the rate of change of y, dy/dt, when $t = 4$?

First, find the rate of change of x, dx/dt:

$$\frac{dx}{dt} = \frac{1}{4\sqrt{t}}.$$

Then

$$\frac{dy}{dx} = 3(x^2 - 1),$$

so that

$$\frac{dy}{dt} = \frac{dx}{dt}\,\frac{dy}{dx}$$

$$= \frac{3(x^2 - 1)}{4\sqrt{t}}$$

when $t = 4$

$$x = \tfrac{1}{2}\sqrt{4} + 3 = 4,$$

and

$$\frac{dy}{dt} = \frac{3(16 - 1)}{(4)2} = \frac{45}{8} \text{ per unit time.}$$

PROBLEM

Water is flowing into the tank as shown below. How fast is it rising?

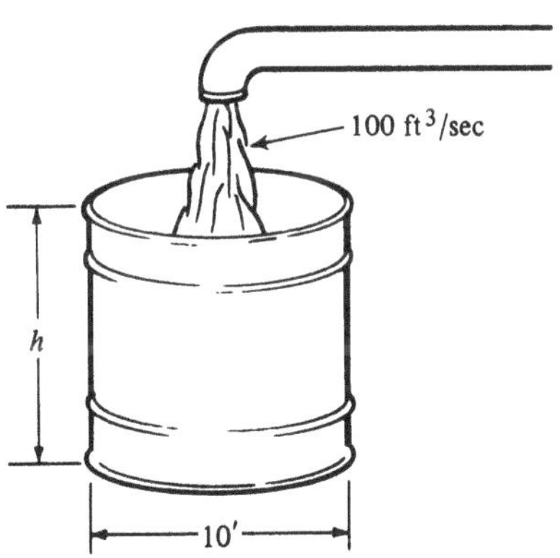

a. 0.3 ft/sec.
b. 1.3 ft/sec.
c. 2.7 ft/sec.
d. 1.8 ft/sec.
e. 0.8 ft/sec.

Check your answer.

Answer

b. $\dfrac{dv}{dt} = 100.$

$$\frac{dh}{dt} = \frac{dv}{dt}\,\frac{dh}{dv}.$$

F. IMPLICIT DIFFERENTIATION

In the previous differentiation problems the functional relationship was first put into the form $y = f(x)$. In this form y is said to be an explicit function of x. In some cases it is difficult or impossible to separate the variables. In such cases, we need a means of differentiating an implicit function such as $y = f(x,y)$. This is done by thinking of each term as a function of x and differentiating term by term.

> In the polynomial
>
> $$C_1x^{n+1} + C_2y^{n+1} = 1$$
>
> implicit differentiation yields
>
> $$(C_1)(n+1)x^n \frac{dx}{dx} + C_2(n+1)y^n \frac{dy}{dx} = 0.$$

Example

$$xy + x - 2y = 1.$$

Differentiating,

$$\frac{xdy}{dx} + \frac{ydx}{dx} + \frac{dx}{dx} - \frac{2dy}{dx} = \frac{d(1)}{dx},$$

or

$$\frac{xdy}{dx} + y + 1 - \frac{2dy}{dx} = 0$$

$$\frac{dy}{dx} = \frac{1+y}{2-x}.$$

If it is desired to find the second derivative of the above expression, we must use implicit differentiation again:

$$\frac{d^2y}{dx^2} = \frac{d(dy/dx)}{dx}$$

$$= \frac{(2-x)\dfrac{dy}{dx} + (1+y)}{4 - 4x + x^2}.$$

The dy/dx term can be eliminated by substituting

$$\frac{dy}{dx} = \frac{1 + y}{2 - x}.$$

Thus,

$$\frac{d^2y}{dx^2} = \frac{2(1 + y)}{4 - 4x + x^2}.$$

PROBLEM

If $2x - 4xy - y = 6$, y' equals:

a. $\dfrac{4y - 2}{4x + 1}$.

b. $\dfrac{2y - 1}{2x + \frac{1}{2}}$.

c. $\dfrac{4y + 2}{-4x - 1}$.

d. $\dfrac{2y - 1}{-2x - \frac{1}{2}}$.

e. None of the above.

Check your answer.

Answer

d.

G. PARTIAL DIFFERENTIATION

Differential calculus is a two-dimensional tool. To use it in three-dimensional space, it is necessary to divide the space into a family of two-dimensional planes.

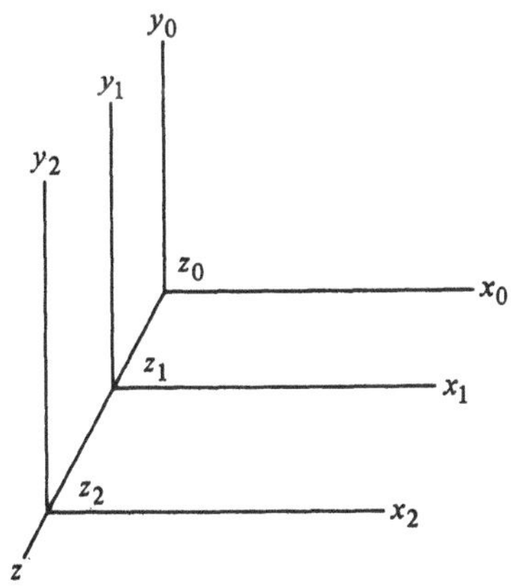

Plane x_1,y_1 is defined by setting $z = z_1$ and holding it constant. In other words, z is no longer a variable. One can then proceed to differentiate as if the problem were in two dimensions.

If $y = f(x,z)$,

$$\left.\frac{\partial y}{\partial x}\right|_z = f'(x,z)$$

$$\left.\frac{\partial y}{\partial z}\right|_x = f'(x,z).$$

Example

$$y = 2zx.$$

Then

$$\left.\frac{\partial y}{\partial x}\right|_z = 2z$$

and

$$\left.\frac{\partial y}{\partial z}\right|_x = 2x.$$

PROBLEM

A plane ($y = 1$) cuts the surface $z = x^2 - 2y^2 - 6$. What is the slope of the resulting line at point (1,1)?

a. $\dfrac{\partial z}{\partial x} = 2.$

b. $\dfrac{\partial x}{\partial z} = 2.$

c. $\dfrac{\partial y}{\partial z} = 2.$

d. $\dfrac{\partial z}{\partial y} = 2.$

e. $\dfrac{\partial x}{\partial y} = 2.$

Check your answer.

Answer

a.
The slope of the line in the x,z plane can be described by either $\partial z/\partial x$ or $\partial x/\partial z$.

H. MAXIMUM AND MINIMUM

A second-degree polynomial can have either a local maximum value or a local minimum value. A third-degree or higher polynomial can have both. These values with respect to the x axis are shown on the following diagram:

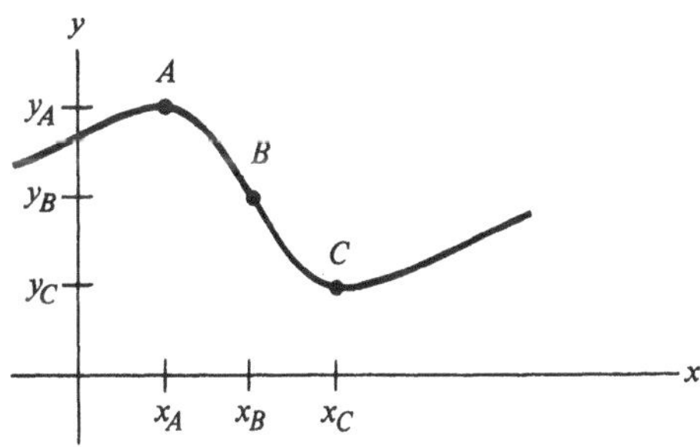

x_A is where the maximum occurs;
y_A is the maximum;
B is the inflection point;
x_C is where the minimum occurs;
y_C is the minimum.
These values are found by the following procedure:

I. The local value of x for $y = f(x)$ at point A (a maximum) can be found by
   a. solving for dy/dx, setting it equal to zero;
   b. solving for d^2y/dx^2 and ascertaining its sign for a value of x found in a. If d^2y/dx^2 is negative, point A is a maximum.

II. The local value of x for point B (an inflection point) is found by finding a value of x which makes $d^2y/dx^2 = 0$.

III. The local value of x for point C (a minimum) is found by setting $dy/dx = 0$. If the second derivative, d^2y/dx^2, is positive, point C is a minimum.

Example

Find the maximum and minimum values of x for the function

$$y = x(12 - 2x)^2.$$

Differentiating,

$$\frac{dy}{dx} = 12(x - 2)(x - 6).$$

Setting dy/dx equal to zero,

$$x = 2 \text{ and } x = 6.$$

The second derivative is

$$\frac{d^2y}{dx^2} = 24(x - 4).$$

Substituting $x = 2$,

$$\frac{d^2y}{dx^2} = 24(2 - 4) = -48;$$

hence $x = 2$ is a maximum. For $x = 6$,

$$\frac{d^2y}{dx^2} = 24(6 - 4) = +48;$$

hence $x = 6$ is a minimum.

PROBLEMS

1. The maximum rectangular area that can be enclosed with 160 ft of fence is:

   a. 3200 ft^2.
   b. 2400 ft^2.
   c. 1600 ft^2.
   d. 1200 ft^2.
   e. 800 ft^2.

2. If $y'' = 0$ at $x = 3$, which of the following is true?

   a. y' is positive.
   b. y' is negative.
   c. The point is a maximum.
   d. The point is a minimum.
   e. None of the above.

Check your answers.

Answers

1. c.
   Derive an expression for $A = f(x)$; then calculate dA/dx and set it equal to zero.
2. e.
   The point is an inflection point. It is the point where y' changes sign.

I. DIFFERENTIATION OF TRIGONOMETRIC FUNCTIONS

Trigonometric functions can be differentiated as well as algebraic functions. A brief table of formulas appears below. Refer to a handbook or a calculus text for a more complete listing of formulas.

Differentiation of Trigonometric Functions:

1. $\frac{d}{dx}(\sin u) = \cos u \frac{du}{dx}$.
2. $\frac{d}{dx}(\cos u) = -\sin u \frac{du}{dx}$.
3. $\frac{d}{dx}(\tan u) = \sec^2 u \frac{du}{dx}$.
4. $\frac{d}{dx}(\cot u) = -\csc^2 u \frac{du}{dx}$.
5. $\frac{d}{dx}(\sec u) = \sec u \tan u \frac{du}{dx}$.
6. $\frac{d}{dx}(\csc u) = -\csc u \cot u \frac{du}{dx}$.

Example

$x = \sin 3\theta$. Then

$$\frac{dx}{d\theta} = 3 \cos 3\theta.$$

PROBLEMS

1. If $f(x) = 2x^2 \cos 2x, f'(x)$ equals:

   a. $2x^2 \sin 2x + 2x \cos 2x$.
   b. $4x(\cos 2x - x \sin 2x)$.
   c. $4 \cos 2x - 4x^2 \sin 2x$.
   d. $4x(\cos x - x \sin x)$.
   e. $2x^2(\cos 2x - \sin 2x)$.

2. The voltage from a generator is given by

$$V = 10 \sin \theta + 4 \sin (90° - \theta),$$

   where θ is the angular position of the rotor. V is maximum when:

   a. $\theta = 0$.
   b. $\sin \theta = 0.5$.
   c. $\cos \theta = 0$.
   d. $\tan \theta = 2.5$.
   e. $\csc \theta = 2$.

Check your answers.

Answers

1. b.
   Use formula 2.
2. d.
   Refer to Section H (maximum and minimum); then use formulas 1 and 2.

J. DIFFERENTIALS

In the first derivative of dy/dx, dy is called the differential of y, and dx is called the differential of x. Since dy/dx derived from $\Delta y/\Delta x$, we can think of the differential as a difference (Δy or Δx). This concept is useful in experimental error analysis. If measured values are variables in a functional relationship, the differentials in the expression for dy/dx represent the experimental tolerances.

> If
>
> $$y = f(x)$$
>
> and
>
> $$\frac{dy}{dx} = f'(x),$$
>
> where x is a measured quantity, then dx is the measurement tolerance and dy is the experimental error in y.

Example

Consider the measurement of the area of a rectangle with a tape measure:

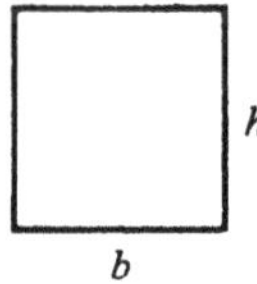

$$A = bh.$$

Experimentally,

$$b = 2 \pm 0.1$$

$$h = 3 \pm 0.1.$$

Implicitly differentiate with respect to an arbitrary variable u:

$$\frac{dA}{du} = \frac{hdb}{du} + \frac{bdh}{du}.$$

Define $du = A$. Then

$$\frac{dA}{A} = \frac{hdb}{hb} + \frac{bdh}{hb} = \frac{db}{b} + \frac{dh}{h}.$$

In the case at hand:

$$A = 2 \times 3 = 6$$

and

$$dA = \frac{6(0.1}{2} + \frac{0.1)}{3} = 0.5.$$

Thus

$$A = 6 \pm 0.5.$$

PROBLEM

The velocity of a bullet passing between two chronograph screens 10 ± 0.1 ft apart with a time interval of 0.01 ± 0.001 sec is:

a. 500 ± 55 ft/sec.
b. 500 ± 49 ft/sec.
c. 1000 ± 105 ft/sec.
d. 1000 ± 99 ft/sec.
e. 1000 ± 110 ft/sec.

Check your answer.

Answer

e.
The tolerance is a plus or minus quantity. Use the combination which yields the worst-case error.

6 Integral Calculus

Discussion of and problems related to the area under a curved line; integration by parts; partial fractions; areas, volumes, and moments; and differential equations.

A. DEFINITIONS

Differentiation, when applied to a single term of a polynomial, results in a reduction of the degree of the polynomial:

If

$$y = x^n$$

then

$$y' = nx^{n-1}.$$

Integration is the reverse of the differentiation operation. Consider the function $y = 2x^2 + 3$:

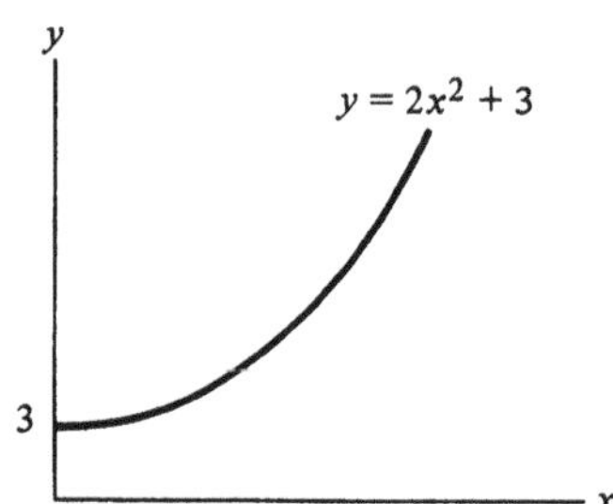

The first derivative is $dy/dx = 4x$ or, plotted:

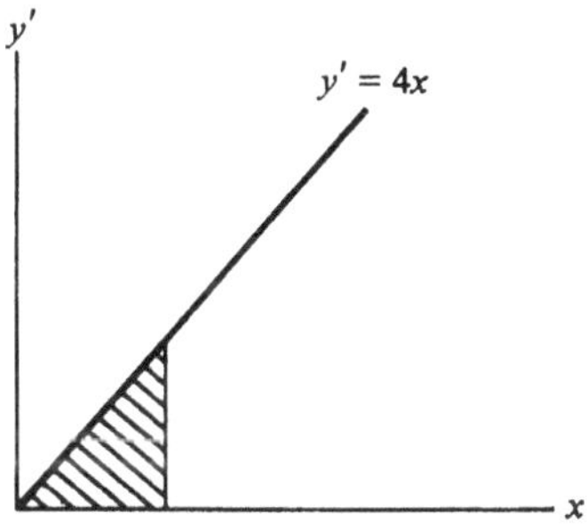

Note the plot of dy/dx and the triangular area under the curve. The area of a triangle is $\frac{1}{2}bh$. In this case, $b = x$ for any value of x, and $h = 4x$, again for any value of x. The area under the curve, then, is

$$A = \tfrac{1}{2}(x)(4x) = 2x^2,$$

which is exactly equal to the first term in the original polynomial,

$$y = 2x^2 + 3.$$

Also note that the area under the curve gives no information about the constant term in the original polynomial (in this case, 3). Because of this, integration is less precise than differentiation.

The preceding concepts can be illustrated symbolically as follows:

If

$$y = f(x)$$

and

$$\frac{dy}{dx} = f'(x),$$

then rearranging produces

$$dy = f'(x)\,dx.$$

The performance of an integration operation is indicated by rewriting the above as

$$y = \int f'(x)\,dx.$$

The solution to the integration operation is

$$y = f(x) + c,$$

where c is an unspecified constant.

Hence, if we differentiate and then integrate, the result is exactly the same as the starting point except that we have added a constant of integration. Determination of this constant of integration is covered in the following example.

Example A

Determine the integral of $y' = 2$, given that the resulting function also passes through point (3,9).

The integration is represented by

$$y = \int 2\,dx.$$

The solution is $y = 2x + c$, where $2x$ is the area under $y' = 2$ for any x. This represents a family of parallel straight lines with slope 2 and y intercept c. If the particular solution must pass through point (3,9), then c can be determined as follows:

$$\begin{aligned} c &= y - 2x \\ &= 9 - 2(3) \\ &= 3, \end{aligned}$$

and the particular solution is

$$y = 2x + 3.$$

Example B

Determine the area under the curve $y' = 2$ between the limits of $x = 1$ and $x = 2$.

This is the definite integral and is written as:

$$y = \int_1^2 2\,dx.$$

The solution is

$$y = 2x\Big|_1^2,$$

which indicates that the function is evaluated between the limits 1 and 2. This evaluation yields

$$y = 2(2) - 2(1) = 2.$$

PROBLEMS

1. If $y = 2x^2 + 3x + 6$, the highest-degree term in the solution of $\int f(x)\,dx$ is:

   a. 4. d. 1.
   b. 3. e. 0.
   c. 2.

2. The area under the curve $y = 3x - 2$ between the limits $x = -2$ and $x = 0$ is:

   a. 4. d. 10.
   b. 6. e. 12.
   c. 8.

Check your answers.

Answers

1. b.
   In the examples presented, observe the change of degree when integrating.
2. d.
   Use the method outlined in Example B, or compute this graphically.

B. AREA UNDER A CURVED LINE

Again, as in differentiation, the integration operation becomes less clear when dealing with curved lines. Consider the area bounded by the function $y = x^2$ and $x = 3$.

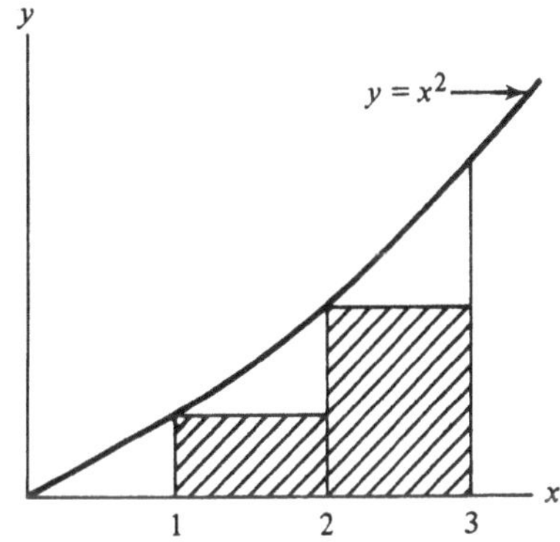

The sum of the shaded rectangles, each Δx units wide and y units high, approximates the total area, but understates it by the amount of the unshaded area. However, as Δx approaches 0, the unshaded area also approaches 0. Therefore, we can say that

$$A = \lim_{\Delta x \to 0} \sum_{0}^{n} y \, \Delta x,.$$

where n is the number of rectangles. In the case at hand, $n = 3/\Delta x$. The sum of the rectangular areas can be evaluated as follows:

$$\begin{aligned} A &= \sum_{0}^{n} y \, \Delta x = \sum_{0}^{n} x^2 \, \Delta x \\ &= x_1^2 \, \Delta x + x_2^2 \, \Delta x + x_3^2 \, \Delta x + \cdots + x_n^2 \, \Delta x. \end{aligned}$$

But from the sketch we see that

$$x_1 = 0, \quad x_2 = \Delta x, \quad x_3 = 2 \, \Delta x, \quad \text{etc.}$$

Thus,

$$\begin{aligned} A &= 0 + (\Delta x)^2 \, \Delta x + (2 \, \Delta x)^2 \, \Delta x + \cdots + [(n - 1) \, \Delta x]^2 \, \Delta x \\ &= [1^2 + 2^2 + \cdots + (n - 1)^2](\Delta x)^3. \end{aligned}$$

By referring to an algebra text we can determine that the sum of the above progression is

$$\tfrac{1}{6}(n - 1)n(2n - 1).$$

Since $\Delta x^3 = (3/n)^3$, we can write the area as the limit of the sum as $n \longrightarrow \infty$ (equivalent to $\Delta x \longrightarrow 0$). This is the definition of the integral:

$$\int y\,dx = \lim_{n\to\infty} \frac{1}{6}(n-1)n(2n-1)\left(\frac{3}{n}\right)^3$$

$$= \lim_{n\to\infty} \frac{9}{2}\,\frac{(n)(2n^2-3n+1)}{n^3}$$

$$= \frac{9}{2}(1)(2) = 9.$$

Inspection shows that 9 is equivalent to $x^3/3$ when $x = 3$. This leads to the general rule:

> If $y = x^n$,
>
> $$\int x^n\,dx = \frac{x^{n+1}}{n+1}.$$

This useful rule holds for any single-term polynomial of the form $y = x^n$. For other integration rules, refer to a calculus text or a handbook.

Example

$y = 2x^3 - x^2$. Evaluate $\int_{-1}^{2} y\,dx$.

$$\int_{-1}^{2} (2x^3 - x^2)\,dx = \frac{2x^4}{4}\Bigg|_{-1}^{2} - \frac{x^3}{3}\Bigg|_{-1}^{2}$$

$$= 8 - \frac{1}{2} - \frac{8}{3} - \frac{1}{3}$$

$$= \frac{9}{2}$$

PROBLEMS

1. $\displaystyle\int \frac{dx}{\sqrt[3]{x^2}}$ equals:

   a. $\frac{2}{3}x^{2/3} + c.$

   b. $3\sqrt[3]{x} + c.$
   c. $x^{-2/3} + c.$

   d. $\frac{2}{3}\sqrt[3]{x} + c.$
   e. None of the above.

2. $\int 3^x \, dx$ equals:

   a. $9^{x+1} + c$.
   b. $3^x + \frac{1}{9} + c$.
   c. $\ln 3^x + c$.
   d. $3^x \ln 3 + c$.
   e. $\dfrac{3^x}{\ln 3} + c$.

Check your answers.

Answers

1. b.
   n in the form $y = x^n$ is $-\frac{2}{3}$. Apply the formula using this value of n.
2. e.
   To work this problem, refer to a text containing a relatively complete set of integration formulas.

C. INTEGRATION BY PARTS

In the previous problem reference was made to a more complete set of integration formulas. In examining such a set, note that the number of formulas is far more extensive than the corresponding differentiation formulas. This is partly because there is no general formula in integration to cover the product or ratio of two functions as there was in differentiation. In other words, no formula covers $\int uv \, dx$, where u and v are functions of x. In such a case one can either find a formula in the extensive tables or use a technique called *integration by parts*.

$$\int u \, dv = uv - \int v \, du.$$

To use:
1. select a part dv that is readily integrable;
2. $\int v \, du$ must not be more complicated than $\int u \, dv$.

Example A

Evaluate

$$\int 3x\sqrt{1 - 2x^2} \, dx.$$

Integration by parts is an appropriate tool in this example, but, on examination, a simpler substitution technique will also work. Let

$$1 - 2x^2 = u.$$

Then differentiate:

$$du = -4x \, dx.$$

Hence,

$$\int 3x\sqrt{u}\,\frac{du}{-4x} = -\frac{3}{4}\int u^{1/2}\,du = -\frac{1}{2}u^{3/2} + c.$$

Substituting back, $u = 1 - 2x^2$, and the answer is

$$-\frac{1}{2}(1 - 2x^2)^{3/2} + c$$

Example B

Evaluate

$$\int x\sqrt{1 + x}\,dx.$$

The simple technique of Example A will not work on this example, so the universal integration by parts formula is used.

Let $u = x$. Then $du = dx$. Let

$$dv = \sqrt{1 + x}\,dx.$$

Then

$$v = \int\sqrt{1 + x}\,dx = \frac{2}{3}(1 + x)^{3/2}.$$

Substituting into the formula,

$$\int x\sqrt{1 + x}\,dx = x\left[\frac{2}{3}(1 + x)^{3/2}\right] - \int\frac{2}{3}(1 + x)^{3/2}\,dx.$$

The remaining integral is in the form x^n, so

$$\int x\sqrt{1 + x}\,dx = x\left[\frac{2}{3}(1 + x)^{3/2}\right] - \frac{4}{15}(1 + x)^{5/2} + c.$$

PROBLEM

Evaluate $\int xe^x\,dx$.

a. $\dfrac{x^2e^x}{2} - e^x + c.$

b. $xe^x - \ln x + c.$

c. $2e^x + c.$

d. $xe^x - e^x + c.$

e. $\dfrac{x^2e^x}{2} - \ln x + c.$

Check your answer.

Answer

d.
Select $u = x$ and $dv = e^x\,dx$. Note how the $\int v\,du$ becomes more complex if the selection $u = e^x$ is made.

D. PARTIAL FRACTIONS

The previous technique, integration by parts, accommodated the case where integration of a product of two functions was desired. *Partial fractions* is a tool to integrate functions in quotient form. This is done by reducing a nonintegrable fraction to a sum of simpler fractions which *are* integrable.

$$\frac{f(x)}{g(x)} = \frac{A}{u(x)} + \frac{B}{u(x)} + \cdots,$$

where $1/u(x)$ is integrable using the formula

$$\int \frac{du}{u} = \ln u + c.$$

Example

Evaluate

$$\int \frac{dx}{x^2 - 4}.$$

Factoring the denominator,

$$x^2 - 4 = (x - 2)(x + 2).$$

Thus,

$$\frac{1}{x^2 - 4} = \frac{A}{x - 2} + \frac{B}{x + 2}.$$

Solving for A and B,

$$\begin{aligned} 1 &= A(x + 2) + B(x - 2) \\ &= (A + B)x + (2A - 2B). \end{aligned}$$

Thus,

$$A + B = 0 \quad \text{and} \quad 2A - 2B = 1.$$

Solving simultaneously,

$$A = \frac{1}{4} \quad \text{and} \quad B = -\frac{1}{4}.$$

Thus,

$$\int \frac{dx}{x^2 - 4} = \frac{1}{4}\int \frac{dx}{x - 2} - \frac{1}{4}\int \frac{dx}{x + 2}$$
$$= \frac{1}{4} \ln \frac{x - 2}{x + 2} + c.$$

PROBLEMS

1. A simpler form of $\dfrac{3x + 5}{x^3 - x^2 - x + 1}$ is:

   a. $\dfrac{2}{x + 1} - \dfrac{2}{x - 1} + \dfrac{1}{4(x - 1)^2}$.
   b. $\dfrac{1}{2}\left(\dfrac{1}{x + 1} - \dfrac{1}{x - 1}\right) + \dfrac{4}{(x - 1)^2}$.
   c. $2\left(\dfrac{1}{x + 1} - \dfrac{1}{x - 1}\right) + \dfrac{2}{(x - 1)^2}$.
   d. $\dfrac{1/2}{x + 1} + \dfrac{1/2}{x - 1} + \dfrac{4}{(x - 1)^2}$.
   e. $\dfrac{1}{2}\left(\dfrac{1}{x^2 - 1}\right) + \dfrac{2}{x - 1}$.

2. What is the most straightforward way to integrate $\displaystyle\int \frac{dx}{\sqrt{1 - x^2}}$?

   a. Maclaurin's series.
   b. Partial fractions.
   c. Handbook of formulas.
   d. L'Hospital's Rule.
   e. Approximation.

Check your answers.

Answers

1. b.
2. c.
   Refer to a handbook of formulas and compare to using partial fractions.

E. AREAS, VOLUMES, AND MOMENTS

Integration yields the area bounded by four lines. The integral $\int_a^b f(x)\,dx$ is defined as the area bounded by the curve $y = f(x)$, the two lines $x = a$ and $x = b$, and the x axis.

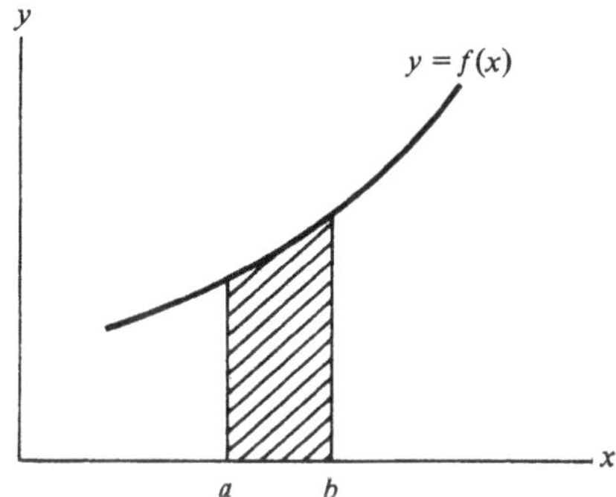

A *volume of revolution* can be defined by displacing an area rotationally
A *moment* is a volume displaced rotationally, multiplied by its radius of rotation.

$$A = \int_a^b f(x)\,dx.$$

$$V = M \int_a^b f(x)\,dx.$$

$$M = M^2 \int_a^b f(x)\,dx.$$

Example

Find the volume of the solid generated by revolving the plane area bounded by the parabola $y^2 = 8x$ and the line $x = 2$ about the x axis.

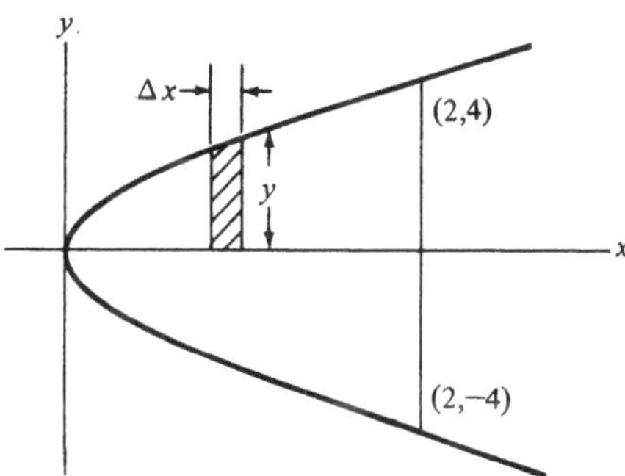

The small rectangle of area $y\ \Delta x$ makes a disk of volume $\pi y^2\ \Delta x$. Thus, the total volume is

$$V = \int_0^2 \pi y^2\,dx = \pi \int_0^2 8x\,dx$$

$$= 4\pi x^2 \Big|_0^2 = 16\pi.$$

PROBLEMS

1. The work done to compress a spring is the area under a force vs. deflection curve. A linear spring with constant $K = 100$ has a normal length of 9 in. How much work is done in stretching it from 10 to 11 in.?

   a. 300 in.-lb.
   b. 75 in.-lb.
   c. 200 in.-lb.
   d. 150 in.-lb.
   e. None of the above.

2. With respect to the cylinder shown below, $\int_0^a x^2(2\pi xb)\,dx$ represents:

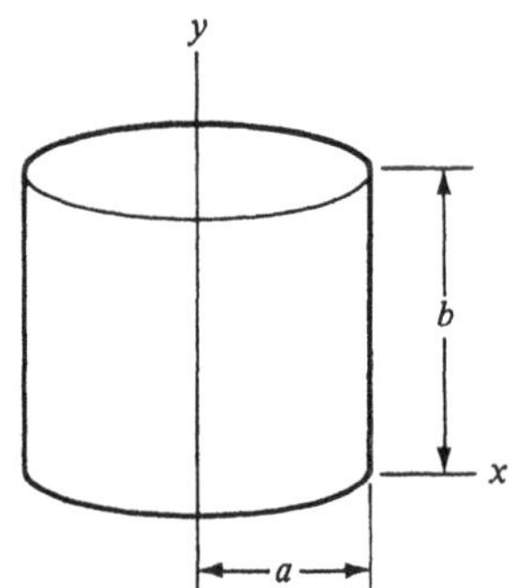

   a. Moment of inertia.
   b. Radius of gyration.
   c. Centroid.
   d. DeMoivre's figure.
   e. Volume.

Check your answers.

Answers

1. d.
   Evaluate $\int_1^2 F\,dx$, where $F = 100x$.
2. a.
   Refer to a textbook definition of moment of inertia.

F. DIFFERENTIAL EQUATIONS

Any algebraic equation containing a derivative is a differential equation. The solution of a differential equation is accomplished by integration. Therefore, this entire chapter deals with the solution of differential equations. The subject bears no further elaboration except when first and second derivatives are involved in an equation. If there is a second derivative, the equation is known as a second-order differential equation.

> A great many of the differential equations found in engineering problems are in the following form:
>
> $$A\frac{d^2x}{dy^2}+B\frac{dx}{dy}+Cx=f(x).$$
>
> In some cases these problems can be solved by defining a *differential operator*:
>
> $$D=\frac{d}{dy}$$
>
> or
>
> $$D^2=\frac{d^2}{dy^2}.$$
>
> Thus, the term Ad^2x/dy^2 is written AD^2x.

After this substitution, the equation is in the form of an ordinary quadratic and can be operated on by the normal methods of algebra, yielding D as a first-order function of x. Substituting back $Dx = dx/dy$ then yields a first-order differential equation, which can be integrated.

Example A

A spring, mass, dash pot system

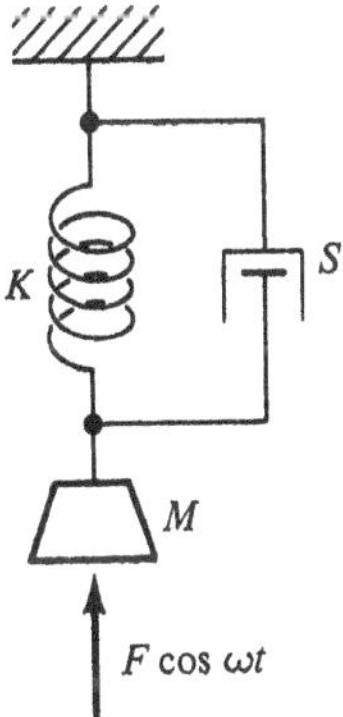

The motion of this system is defined by

$$\frac{Md^2y}{dt}+\frac{S\,dy}{dt}+Ky=F\cos\omega t.$$

Note that each term of the equation has the units of force. Inserting the differential operator $d/dt = D$,

$$MD^2y+SDy+Ky=F\cos\omega t$$

$$y(MD^2+SD+K)=F\cos\omega t.$$

A complete solution of the above equation is quite complex. Usually a system such as the above is solved only for specific conditions.

Consider the case where the system is undamped ($S = 0$) and where no forcing function exists. The resulting differential equation is

$$\frac{M\,d^2y}{dt^2} + Ky = 0.$$

What would be the frequency of oscillation if the mass is displaced from equilibrium and then released?

Applying the differential operator $Dy = dy/dt$ yields

$$MD^2y + Ky = 0$$

or

$$y(MD^2 + K) = 0.$$

Therefore $MD^2 + K = 0$, or

$$D = \pm\sqrt{\frac{K}{M}}.$$

Since $Dy = dy/dt$,

$$D = \frac{dy}{dt/y} = \text{frequency}$$

because velocity and frequency of cyclical motion are related as: $V = \omega r$. Therefore,

$$\omega = \sqrt{\frac{K}{M}}.$$

This is called the natural frequency of oscillation of an undamped spring.

Example B

The foregoing solution can also be applied to an electrical circuit containing resistors, inductors, and capacitors.

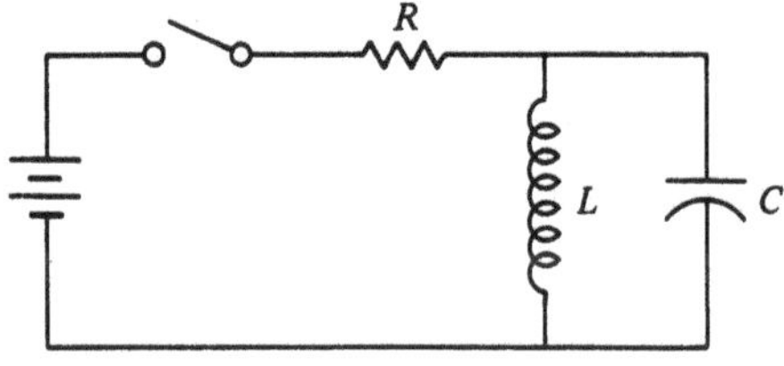

The current in this circuit is governed by the equation

$$L\frac{d^2q}{dt^2} + R\frac{dq}{dt} + \frac{1}{C}q = F(t).$$

Note that each term has the units of voltage. An analagous solution with $F(t) = 0$ and $R = 0$ yields the resonant frequency of an undamped circuit.

PROBLEMS

1. The differential equation

$$\frac{dy}{dx} = \frac{-x}{y}$$

represents a:

a. Circle.
b. Parabola.
c. Ellipse.
d. Moment.
e. Centroid.

2. The resonant frequency in Hz of an electric circuit is given by:

a. $\sqrt{\frac{1}{LC}}$.
b. $\sqrt{\frac{2\pi}{LC}}$.
c. $\sqrt{\frac{C}{L}}$.
d. $\frac{1}{2\pi\sqrt{LC}}$.
e. $\frac{2\pi}{\sqrt{LC}}$.

Check your answers.

Answers

1. a.
   A solution of this equation is $x^2 + y^2 = c$.
2. d.
   Solve the equation of Example B using the methods of Example A.

7 Wave Theory

Discussion of and problems related to the Doppler Effect and refraction.

A. APPLICATION

Electromagnetic radiation such as light or radio and harmonic sound are propagated in the form of sinusoidal waves.

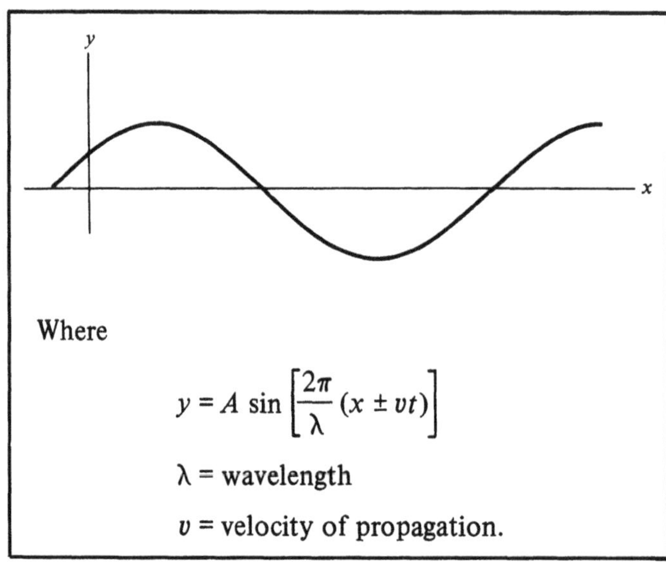

Example

What is the pitch or frequency of sound waves having a wavelength of 100 mm?

Frequency is defined as $f = v/\lambda$. The velocity of sound in air is approximately 300 m/s. Therefore:

$$f = \frac{300}{0.1} = 3000 \text{ Hz.}$$

PROBLEMS

1. Monochromatic light with wavelength 6×10^3 Å has a frequency of:

   a. 500,000 MHz.
   b. 300,000 kHz.
   c. 500,000 GHz.
   d. 300,000 MHz.
   e. 500,000 kHz.

2. The intensity of sound in decibels is

$$\text{dB} = 10 \log \left(\frac{I}{I_0}\right),$$

where $I_0 = 10^{-16}$ W/cm^2.

What is the intensity of two 70-dB sound sources?

   a. 70 dB.
   b. 73 dB.
   c. 78 dB.
   d. 105 dB.
   e. 140 dB.

Check your answers.

Answers

1. c.
   Convert Å to m. Use $v = 3 \times 10^8$ m/s.
2. b.
   $I = 10^7$ for 70 dB.

$$10 \log 2 \times 10^7 = 73.$$

B. DOPPLER EFFECT

If a sound receiver is moving toward or away from a sound emitter, use the relative velocity in the frequency equation. This causes an apparent shift in frequency.

Perceived frequency is
$$f' = \frac{f}{1 \pm v/c},$$
where
v = receiver velocity
c = speed of sound.

Example

A locomotive is traveling at 50 mph and blowing its whistle at 500 Hz. As it comes toward us,

$$f' = \frac{500}{1 - \frac{50}{716}} = 538 \text{ Hz},$$

and as it goes away,

$$f' = \frac{500}{1 + \frac{50}{716}} = 467 \text{ Hz}.$$

PROBLEMS

1. If $c = \sqrt{\frac{\gamma p}{\rho}}$ where $\gamma = 1.4$ for air, what is the velocity of sound nearest to when the barometer reads 28.5 in. Hg and the thermometer reads 40°F?

   a. 1000 ft/sec.
   b. 1050 ft/sec.
   c. 1100 ft/sec.
   d. 1150 ft/sec.
   e. 1200 ft/sec.

2. How fast must one drive to make the car-horn pitch 10% higher? (Use c = 716 mph.)

   a. 45 mph.
   b. 50 mph.
   c. 55 mph.
   d. 60 mph.
   e. 65 mph.

Check your answers.

Answers

1. c.
   The density of air under these conditions is 0.0755 lb/ft^3. If you had difficulty with this problem, do a careful units check.
2. e.
   Solve for $v/716$ such that $f' = (1.1)f$.

C. REFRACTION

Snell's law represents sound or light as a plane front. If this plane front is incident on a material of differing speed of propagation, the rays will be refracted.

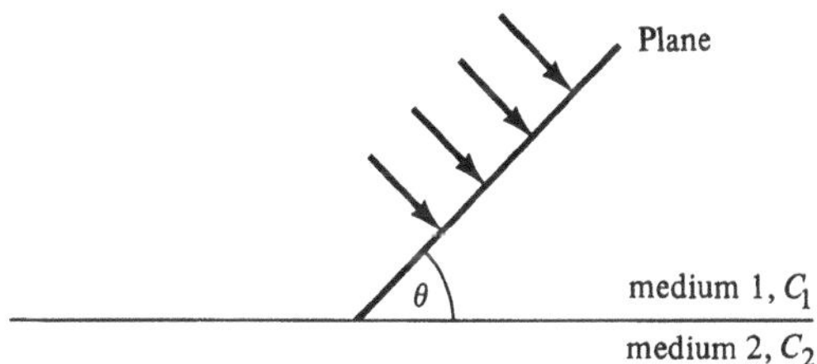

If $C_2 < C_1$, the bottom of the plane will slow down before the top, which refracts the rays closer to normal. If $C_2 > C_1$, the opposite is true.

Snell's Law:

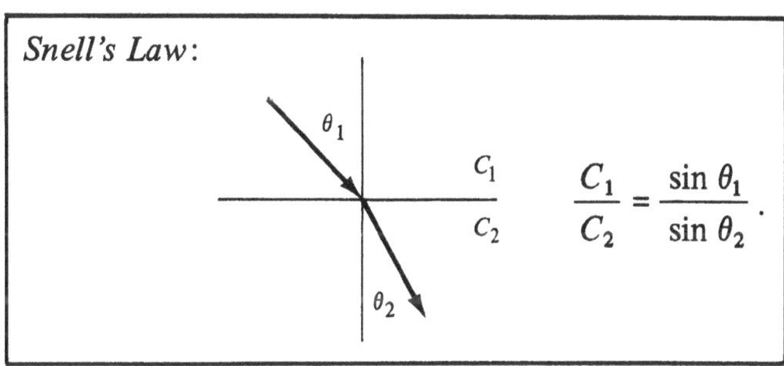

$$\frac{C_1}{C_2} = \frac{\sin\theta_1}{\sin\theta_2}.$$

Example

A man is looking at an angle of 45° at the surface of a pond. At what angle is he actually viewing the fish?

$$C_{air} = 3 \times 10^8 \text{ m/s}.$$

$$C_{water} = 2.2 \times 10^8 \text{ m/s}.$$

$$\sin\theta = \sin 45^\circ \frac{2.20}{3.00}.$$

$$\sin\theta = 0.707 \frac{2.20}{3.00} = 0.518$$

$$\theta = 31^\circ.$$

PROBLEM

The index of refraction for glass is 1.5. At what angle of incidence will the glass appear to reflect all light?

a. 41°.
b. 49°.
c. 62°.
d. 68°.
e. 74°.

Check your answer.

Answer

a.
Set $\theta_2 = 90°$. You may wish to review the definition of index of refraction if you had difficulty with this problem.

8 Chemistry

Discussion of and problems related to atomic theory, the periodic table, molecules, the reaction equation, chemical weights, oxidation-reduction, acid-base neutralization, solutions, and electrolysis.

A. ATOMIC THEORY

In the 1800s Dalton postulated the existence of the atom. According to Dalton's atomic theory, atoms were:

- undivisible,
- unchangeable,
- peculiar to each element.

In other words, the smallest particle of an element like copper is the copper atom which cannot be created, destroyed, or changed and which, further, is unlike the atom of any other element.

Later, in the 1920s, Bohr developed an atomic model consisting of a massive nucleus containing positively charged protons and electrically neutral neutrons surrounded by orbiting negatively charged electrons.

The atom in the Bohr model is held together by electrostatic forces. Graphically, the electrons of a heavy element occupy orbits as shown at top of p. 88.

The atom of a particular element can be identified by two numbers:

1. the atomic number—the number of charged particles, either electrons or protons;
2. the atomic weight—the number of nuclear particles (protons and neutrons).

Table 1 lists the atomic numbers and atomic weights for the more common elements.

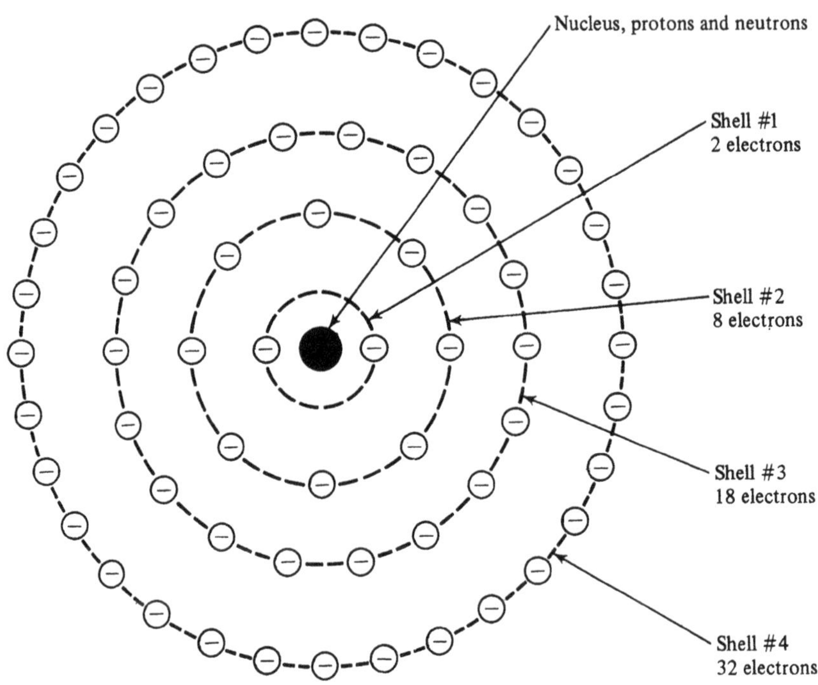

Table 1. Atomic Numbers and Weights for Common Chemical Elements

Element	Symbol	Atomic Number	Atomic Weight	Element	Symbol	Atomic Number	Atomic Weight
Aluminum	Al	13	26.97	Lead	Pb	82	207.21
Argon	Ar	18	39.944	Lithium	Li	3	6.940
Arsenic	As	33	74.91	Magnesium	Mg	12	24.32
Barium	Ba	56	137.36	Manganese	Mn	25	54.93
Beryllium	Be	4	9.02	Mercury	Hg	80	200.61
Bismuth	Bi	83	209.00	Molybdenum	Mo	42	95.95
Boron	B	5	10.82	Neon	Ne	10	20.183
Bromine	Br	35	79.916	Nickel	Ni	28	58.69
Cadmium	Cd	48	112.41	Nitrogen	N	7	14.008
Calcium	Ca	20	40.08	Oxygen	O	8	16.0000
Carbon	C	6	12.010	Phosphorus	P	15	30.98
Cesium	Cs	55	132.91	Platinum	Pt	78	195.23
Chlorine	Cl	17	35.457	Potassium	K	19	39.096
Chromium	Cr	24	52.01	Selenium	Se	34	78.96
Cobalt	Co	27	58.94	Silicon	Si	14	28.06
Copper	Cu	29	63.54	Silver	Ag	47	107.880
Fluorine	F	9	19.00	Sodium	Na	11	22.997
Gold	Au	79	197.2	Sulfur	S	16	32.066
Helium	He	2	4.003	Tin	Sn	50	118.70
Hydrogen	H	1	1.0080	Titanium	Ti	22	47.90
Iodine	I	53	126.92	Tungsten	W	74	183.92
Iron	Fe	26	55.85	Uranium	U	92	238.07
Krypton	Kr	36	83.7	Zinc	Zn	30	65.38

Bohr Atomic Model:
a. The atom is made up of a nucleus and rings of electrons.
b. Each electron has a negative electrical charge.
c. The nucleus contains positively charged particles called protons equal in number to the number of electrons.
d. The nucleus also contains noncharged particles approximately equal in number to the protons.
e. The number of protons in the nucleus is the atomic number of the element.
f. The mass of the electrons is very small, and the mass of the protons and neutrons are both equal to one atomic weight.

Example

Using the preceding table, the helium atom may be described as having an atomic number of 2 and an atomic weight of 4.* Symbolically the atom can be described as: ${}_2He^4$. Graphically it is represented as follows:

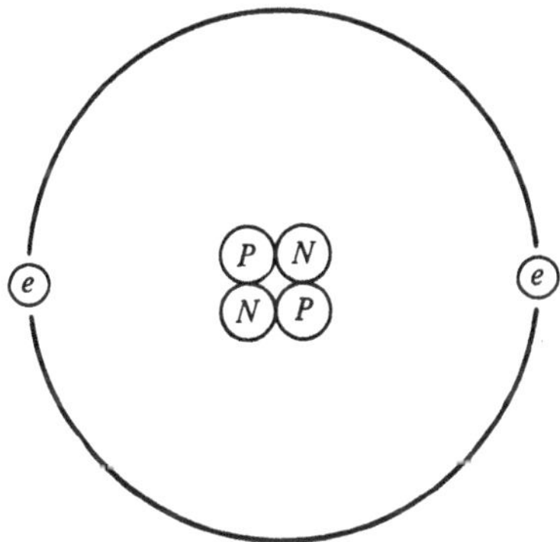

PROBLEMS

1. The most commonly occurring isotope of aluminum has how many neutrons in its nucleus?

   a. 13.   d. 15.
   b. 14.   e. 12.
   c. 27.

2. Approximately what percentage of carbon in nature is carbon 13?

   a. 0.01%.   d. 10%.
   b. 0.10%.   e. None of the above.
   c. 1.0%.

Check your answers.

*Actually 4.003. This happens because there are some naturally occurring "isotopes" of helium with an extra neutron in the nucleus.

Answers

1. b.
   Atomic weight less the number of protons.
2. c.
   One carbon 13 per 100 carbon 12.

B. THE PERIODIC TABLE

Progressively heavier elements can be visualized by systematically adding one proton at a time. For every proton added, an electron is also added. When an electron orbit is full, a new orbit is started. This gives a periodic aspect to arranging the elements in a matrix–hence the periodic table for the more common elements (Table 2).

Table 2. Periodic Table for the More Common Elements.

	Metals												Nonmetals					
Group	I	II											III	IV	V	VI	VII	O
Period I	H 1																	He 2
Period II	Li 3	Be 4											B 5	C 6	N 7	O 8	F 9	Ne 10
Period III	Na 11	Mg 12	Transition Metals										Al 13	Si 14	P 15	S 16	Cl 17	A 18
Period IV	K 19	Ca 20	Sc 21	Ti 22	V 23	Cr 24	Mn 25	Fe 26	Co 27	Ni 28	Cu 29	Zn 30	Ga 31	Ge 32	As 33	Se 34	Br 35	Kr 36
Period V	Rb 37	Sr 38	Y 39	Zr 40	Nb 41	Mo 42	Tc 43	Ru 44	Rh 45	Pd 46	Ag 47	Cd 48	In 49	Sn 50	Sb 51	Te 52	I 53	Xe 54
Period VI	Cs 55	Ba 56				W 74					Au 79	Hg 80	Tl 81	Pb 82	Bi 83	Po 84	At 85	Rn 86

Note that each column represents the same number of electrons in the outer orbit, and each row represents the number of orbits. The elements in group 0 (helium, neon, argon, etc.) are all totally inert. They also each have 8 electrons in their outer orbit, with the exception of helium, which has 2. This means that a full outer orbit is 8 electrons (or 2 for helium) and that a full outer orbit represents chemical stability.

Elements in the other groups will tend to acquire or to give up electrons to achieve a full outer orbit. Those on the left will give up electrons; those on the right will acquire; those in the center may do either.

When an atom has other than the correct number of electrons, it is a charged particle called an *ion*. The amount of this charge is called the *valence number*.

> A full outer shell is 8 electrons (2 for Period I).
>
> The charge associated with achieving a full outer shell is the valence number.

Example

The electron distribution and valence for selenium is as follows:

$_{34}Se^{79}$

1st shell 2
2nd shell 8
3rd shell 18
4th shell 6

If the selenium atom acquires 2 more electrons for stability, it will be negatively charged; therefore, the valence number is -2.

PROBLEMS

1. How many electrons are in the fourth shell for potassium?

   a. 2. d. 1.
   b. 8. e. 3.
   c. 18.

2. What valence number(s) should phosphorus have?

   a. +3. d. -3, +5.
   b. -3, +3. e. -5.
   c. -5, +3.

Check your answers.

Answers

1. d.
2. d.

C. MOLECULES

Completely inert elements have an outer shell of either 2 electrons (helium) or 8 electrons. All chemical bonding of elements to form molecules results from the interaction of electrons in the outer shell. There is always a tendency to achieve a stable number of electrons in the outer shell, either 2 (in the case of hydrogen only) or 8. These outer-shell electrons are called the *valence electrons.*

Covalent Bond

The covalent bond is the bonding mechanism that occurs when two or more atoms have the same or similar valence shell. By sharing some of their valence electrons, they can each be in a stable configuration. For example, nitrogen has a total of 7 electrons: 2 in the first shell, 5 in the outer shell. Two nitrogen atoms form a covalent bond by sharing 3 of these outer 5 with each other.

Symbolically this may be represented as follows:

:N⋮⋮N:

This is the molecule N_2, held together by a very strong bond. Free nitrogen always assumes the N_2 molecular bond. Oxygen and hydrogen also occur in nature as the diatomic molecules O_2 and H_2.

Ionic Bond

The chemical formula shows the atomic makeup of the molecule. For example, H_2O. The elements H and O are combined through chemical bonding. The chemical combining capacity, or valence, of an atom is determined by the number of outermost electrons that take part in the bond.

A covalent bond involves ions of like sign which share electrons.
An ionic bond is electrostatic force between ions of opposite sign.

Example

The barium phosphate bond illustrates the process of bonding.

A positive ion is an atom that is missing electrons (positive valence). A negative ion has surplus electrons.

- Barium phosphate is $Ba_3\,(PO_4)_2$.
- Ba has a +2 valence–positive ion.
- PO_4 has a -3 valence–negative ion.

Within the phosphate radical (PO_4),

- O has a -2 valence;
- P has a +5 valence.

Note that phosphate is bivalent because of its near-center position in the periodic table. Its valence here can be inferred from the bond with oxygen.

PROBLEMS

1. Borax is $Na_2B_4O_7$. The valence of boron is:

   a. -5.
   b. +12.
   c. +2.
   d. -3.
   e. +3.

2. The molecular weight of borax is:

   a. 49
   b. 50
   c. 201
   d. 202
   e. 146

Check your answers.

Answers

1. e.
2. c.

D. THE REACTION EQUATION

Consider the disassociation of water to form oxygen and hydrogen:

$$2H_2O \longrightarrow 2H_2 + O_2.$$

The equation is balanced since the same number of atoms of each type appear on both sides of the arrow. From a balanced reaction equation, certain calculations can be made. For example, we can say that two molecules of water disassociate to form two molecules of diatomic hydrogen and one molecule of diatomic oxygen. A more practical unit of measure is the mole which allows the conversion of atomic weight into practical weight units.

$$\text{Avogadro's number} = 6.02 \times 10^{23} \text{ molecules/mole.}$$

1 mole is a quantity which has a weight in grams equal to the molecular weight.

$$n = \frac{w}{mw} \quad \text{or} \quad n = \frac{w}{aw},$$

where

n = number of moles
w = weight in grams
mw = molecular weight
aw = atomic weight.

Example A

80.16 grams of calcium is used in a reaction. How many moles are involved?

$$\frac{80.16 \text{ grams}}{40.08 \text{ grams/mole}} = 2.0 \text{ moles.}$$

Example B

Electrolysis of water produces two moles of hydrogen for each two moles of water.

PROBLEMS

1. In the electrolysis of water, how many grams of H_2O will yield 96 grams of oxygen (O_2)?

   a. 54. d. 32.
   b. 96. e. 108.
   c. 216.

2. How many pounds of calcium carbonate are needed to make 22 lb of glass ($Na_2O \cdot CaO \cdot 7SiO_2$) if the other constituents used are Na_2CO_3 and SiO_2?

   a. 4. d. 10.
   b. 3. e. 5.
   c. 6.

Check your answers.

Answers

1. e.
2. a.
   Calcium carbonate is $CaCO_3$.

E. OXIDATION-REDUCTION

The term *oxidation* was originally applied to reactions where oxygen is added to a compound; reduction was applied to reactions where it is removed. For every oxidation there must be a corresponding reduction in the same reaction.

The present definition of an oxidation-reduction (redox) reaction involves the corresponding changes in valence, with no requirement that oxygen be involved.

The material that is oxidized becomes more positive. The material that is reduced becomes more negative.

Example

$$Fe_2O_3 + 3H_2 \longrightarrow Fe + 3H_2O.$$

Fe is reduced.
H_2 is oxidized.

In this example, the valence of Fe became more negative than it was before the reaction, while the valence of H became more positive.

PROBLEMS

1. In the previous example, the valence change of iron is:

   a. 6.
   b. 10.
   c. 3.
   d. 5.
   e. 2.

2. Three grams of carbon are burned using seven grams of oxygen. The products are carbon dioxide and carbon monoxide. What fraction is CO_2?

   a. 3/8.
   b. 3/4.
   c. 1/2.
   d. 2/3.
   e. 7/8.

Check your answers.

Answers

1. c.
2. b.

F. ACID-BASE NEUTRALIZATION

Hydrogen ions from the acid combine with hydroxide ions from the base, forming water and a salt. In the following complete reaction,

$$H_2SO_4 + 2NaOH \longrightarrow 2H_2O + Na_2SO_4,$$

one mole of sulfuric acid is completely neutralized by two moles of sodium hydroxide.

Most such acid-base reactions involve solutions of the acids and bases in water. To facilitate calculating the exact proportions which will result in a complete reaction, the concept of *normality* has been developed. A one-normal ($1N$) solution contains one gram equivalent weight per liter of water. The gram equivalent weight is the molecular weight divided by the number of hydrogen or hydroxide ions per molecule dissociated in solution.

$$EW = \frac{MW}{H^+ \text{ or } (OH)^-}$$

$$1N = \frac{1 \text{ EW}}{\text{liter}}.$$

Equal volumes of acids and bases of equal normality will exactly neutralize each other.

Normality is a way of stating the strength of an acid or basic solution. Another way is a measure called pH (parts hydrogen), based on the fact that pure water contains some hydrogen and hydroxide ions that are dissociated but in equilibrium. To be exact, pure water contains 10^{-7} moles per liter of these ions. When an acid is added to the water, the H^+ ions will increase. When a base is added, the $(OH)^-$ ions will increase. Some of them will combine with the H^+, causing a decrease in the H^+ ion concentration.

$$pH = \log \frac{1}{[H^+]}.$$

$[H^+]$ is the concentration of hydrogen ions in moles per liter.

$0 < pH < 7$ is an acid.

$pH > 7$ is a base.

Example A

In the sulfuric acid–sodium hydroxide reaction,

$$H_2SO_4 + 2NaOH \longrightarrow 2H_2O + Na_2SO_4,$$

1 EW of H_2SO_4 = 98/2 = 49. Therefore, a 1N solution consists of 49 grams per liter. This will exactly neutralize 500 ml of 2N NaOH.

Example B

What is the pH of a solution found to have 10^{-6} moles of H^+ ions per liter?

$$pH = \log \frac{1}{10^{-6}} = \log 10^6 = 6.$$

This defines the solution as an acid.

PROBLEMS

1. How many grams of hydrogen sulfate (H_2SO_4) mixed with 2000 cc of water will make a 3N solution?

   a. 588. d. 294.
   b. 147. e. 49.
   c. 98.

2. How many milliliters of 0.5N H_2SO_4 will neutralize 0.5 liter of 0.2N NaOH?

   a. 200. d. 300.
   b. 100. e. 600.
   c. 400.

Check your answers.

Answers

1. d.
2. a.

G. SOLUTIONS

The strength of any solution can be stated in terms of *molarity*. A one molar solution contains one molecular weight of solute per liter of solution. A one-molar ($1M$) solution will depress the freezing point 1.86°C below that of pure water.

$$1M = \frac{1 \text{ MW solute}}{\text{liter solution}}.$$

Example A

How much sugar is in a $1M$ solution?

Sugar is $C_{12}H_{22}O_{11}$. Its molecular weight is 342.3. Thus, a $1M$ solution contains 342.3 grams of sugar.

Example B

What is the freezing point of a solution containing 1.027 kg of sugar per liter?

$$\text{molarity} = \frac{1027}{342} = 3.$$

$$\text{Freezing point} = 0 - (3)(1.86) = 5.6°\text{C}.$$

PROBLEM

If 1.6 grams of solute in 150 cc of water freezes at -0.11°C, what is the molecular weight of the solute?

a. 90.
b. 270.
c. 180.
d. 225.
e. 135.

Check your answer.

Answer

c.

H. ELECTROLYSIS

Energy is either released when a reaction occurs (exothermic reaction), or it must be applied to get the reaction to occur (endothermic reaction).

In the case of an endothermic decomposition reaction, the most usual way of causing the reaction is to pass an electric current through the material. The disassociation is called electrolysis. The basic unit of material dissociated is an equivalent weight (EW). Some materials electrolyzed do not have hydrogen ions, so we define an EW as the molecular weight divided by the valence change. This is possible because the H^+ ion has a valence change of one unit.

Faraday's Law:
For each EW of material transferred, 6.02×10^{23} electrons must flow through the circuit.

$$1 \text{ farad} = 6.02 \times 10^{23} \text{ electrons}$$

$$= 96{,}500 \text{ coulombs}$$

$$1 \text{ coulomb} = 1 \text{ amp per second}$$

$$1 \text{ EW} = \text{MW/valence change}$$

Example

In the electrolysis of sodium chloride to produce sodium, how much electricity is required to produce 46 grams?

$$\text{MW} = 23 = \text{EW}$$

$$46 \text{ grams} = 2 \text{ MW}.$$

Since Na^+ has a valence of 1,

$$Na^+\bar{Cl} \longrightarrow Na + Cl.$$

Thus 2 farads are required.

PROBLEM

In a copper-plating process using copper sulfate ($CuSO_4$), what is the hourly rate of deposit with a 10 amp current?

a. 23.6.
b. 5.9.
c. 9.8.
d. 11.8.
e. 35.4.

Check your answer.

Answer

d.

9 Gas Laws

Discussion of and problems related to the Perfect Gas Law and changes of state.

A. THE PERFECT GAS LAW

Gases at relatively low density approximately obey the perfect or ideal gas law. The perfect gas law is a relationship of the measurable parameters: pressure, temperature, and volume.

Perfect Gas Law:

$$pV = nRT$$

where

p = pressure, psfa;
V = volume, cubic feet;
n = lb-moles;
R = universal gas constant (1546);
T = temperature, degrees Rankine.

Example

The pressure of one mole of an ideal gas occupying 40 ft^3 at a temperature of 100°F is expressed as follows:

$$p = \frac{nRT}{V} = \frac{(1)(1546)(100 + 460)}{40}$$

$$= 21644 \text{ psfa}$$

$$= 150.3 \text{ psia.}$$

PROBLEMS

1. How many molecules of gas will occupy 387 ft^3 at room ambient conditions?

   a. 2.52×10^{18}.
   b. 6.02×10^{23}.
   c. 2.73×10^{26}.
   d. 1.84×10^{9}.
   e. 3.29×10^{-24}.

2. The density of diatomic oxygen in a 5 ft^3 container at 140°F and 50 psig is:

   a. 0.14 lb/ft^3.
   b. 0.01 lb/ft^3.
   c. 0.25 lb/ft^3.
   d. 0.16 lb/ft^3.
   e. 0.32 lb/ft^3.

Check your answers.

Answers

1. c.
   Use 14.7 psia and 68°F for room ambient conditions.

$$N = \frac{PV}{RT} = \frac{(14.7)(144)(387)}{1546(528)}$$

$$= 1.004$$

2. e.

B. CHANGES OF STATE

The perfect gas law is useful in determining the changes in properties (pressure, temperature, or volume) when a gas undergoes a change from one state to another.

> Since $pV/nT = R$, the universal gas constant, a process from state 1 to state 2 can be written:
>
> $$\frac{p_1 V_1}{n_1 T_1} = \frac{p_2 V_2}{n_2 T_2}.$$

Example

An oxygen cylinder with an internal volume of 3 cubic feet is initially at 1000 psig and 80°F. When a certain amount of gas is used from the cylinder, both the pressure and temperature drop to 800 psig and 70°F, respectively. How much oxygen was used?

Assume state 1 is prior to use and state 2 is after use. Then

$$\frac{p_1 V_1}{n_1 T_1} = \frac{p_2 V_2}{n_2 T_2},$$

or, since $V_1 = V_2$,

$$\frac{n_2}{n_1} = \frac{p_2}{p_1} \cdot \frac{T_1}{T_2} = \frac{815}{1015} \cdot \frac{540}{530} = 0.82,$$

meaning that 18% of the initial oxygen was used.

In terms of weight,

$$\text{w} = n_1(\text{mw})(0.18)$$

where

w = weight in lb

mw = molecular weight of oxygen

and

$$n_1 = \frac{p_1 V_1}{R T_1}.$$

Therefore,

$$\text{w} = \frac{(1015)(144)(3)}{(1546)(540)}(32)(0.18) = 3 \text{ lb}.$$

PROBLEMS

1. A tank of nitrogen at 400 psig and 70°F is purged until the pressure is 200 psig at 70°F. What weight percentage was purged?

   a. 48.2.
   b. 51.8.
   c. 50.
   d. 49.
   e. 51.

2. In the above tank, the purged nitrogen occupies 600 ft^3 at 50°F and 14.7 psia. What is the volume of the tank?

   a. 61.7 ft^3
   b. 55.2 ft^3
   c. 40.7 ft^3
   d. 45.8 ft^3
   e. 48.2 ft^3

Check your answers.

Answers

1. a.
2. d.

Part II Engineering Fundamentals

The material covered in Part II of this book concentrates on the engineering fundamentals which are included in the curriculum of an accredited engineering school. This material will appear in both the morning and afternoon session of the National Examination. The organization of the text material is the same as Part I, consisting of short multiple-choice questions similar to those in the morning session of the examination.

The afternoon session of the examination consists of problem situations with ten multiple-choice questions associated with each situation. Accordingly, each chapter of Part II concludes with a set of questions similar in format and content to those which will be presented in the afternoon session of the examination.

10 Combustion

Discussion of and problems related to stoichiometric combustion of hydrocarbons and combustion in air.

A. INTRODUCTION

Combustion is an exothermic reaction between a fuel and an oxidant. The simplest combustion reaction is the hydrogen–oxygen reaction. The chemical coefficient can be read as molar quantities or converted to mass quantities using the molecular weight. With gaseous fuel it may be more convenient to work with volumetric quantities. In this case, the ideal gas laws show that if pressure and temperature of the reactants are the same, then the molar ratios can be read as volumetric ratios.

In the reaction

$$2H_2 + O_2 \longrightarrow 2H_2O$$

we can say:

- 2 moles of diatomic hydrogen react with 1 mole of diatomic oxygen to form 2 moles of water.
- 4 lb of hydrogen react with 32 lb of oxygen to form 36 lb of water (since atomic weights for hydrogen and oxygen equal 1 and 16, respectively).
- 2 ft^3 of hydrogen react with 1 ft^3 of oxygen. (Note that we cannot extend the ideal gas law assumption from the reactants to the products since temperature and pressure are not the same.)

Example

Carbon is burned in oxygen with the following incomplete reaction:

$$8C + 7O_2 \longrightarrow 2CO + 6CO_2.$$

We can achieve this reaction by using:

$$(8)(12) = 96 \text{ lb carbon}$$

and

$$(7)(32) = 224 \text{ lb oxygen}$$

and we can say that in the products we have 3 ft^3 of CO_2 for each 4 ft^3 of products.

PROBLEMS

1. An Orsat analysis of flue gases indicates the following volumetric analysis:

$$CO_2 = 13\%$$
$$O_2 = 7\%$$
$$N_2 = 80\%.$$

What is the percent nitrogen by weight?

a. 28.
b. 74.
c. 22.4.
d. 30.4.
e. 82.

2. When nitroglycerin $C_3H_5(NO_3)_3$ reacts, it forms CO_2, H_2O, N_2, and O_2. What is the volumetric ratio of carbon dioxide to oxygen?

a. 2.
b. 6.
c. 12.
d. 3.
e. 14.

Check your answers.

Answers

1. b.
An Orsat analysis is a volumetric analysis. You should be prepared to look up terms such as this during the examination.
2. c.

B. STOICHIOMETRIC COMBUSTION OF HYDROCARBONS

A stoichiometric reaction is one in which all of the fuel and oxygen take part in the reaction. Hydrocarbon fuels consist of a whole family of organic CH molecules which can be gaseous, liquid, or solid.

> The Stoichiometric Hydrocarbon Reaction:
>
> $$AC_xH_y + BO_2 \longrightarrow CCO_2 + DH_2O,$$
>
> where x and y are integers for a pure hydrocarbon but are not necessarily integers for mixtures of hydrocarbons.

Example

Gasoline can be approximated by octane (C_8H_{18}). The stochiometric reaction is:

$$C_8H_{18} + 12.5O_2 \longrightarrow 8CO_2 + 9H_2O.$$

We can reach such conclusions as:

- 12.5 ft^3 of O_2 reacts with 1 ft^3 of fuel.
- There are 1.42 lb of water in the products per lb of fuel.

PROBLEMS

1. Propane (C_3H_8) reacts stochiometrically with oxygen. What is the volumetric ratio of oxygen to fuel?

   a. 20.
   b. 4.
   c. 3.
   d. 12.
   e. 5.

2. Methane is burned with less than stochiometric oxygen. The products could contain which of the following?

   a. CH_4, C, CO_2, H_2O.
   b. C_3H_6C, CO, CO_2, H_2O.
   c. CH_4, C, CO, CO_2, H_2O.
   d. C_3H_6, CO, CO_2, H_2O.
   e. CH_4, CO_2, H_2O.

Check your answers.

Answers

1. e.
2. c.

C. COMBUSTION IN AIR

Air is a mixture of oxygen and nitrogen. The nitrogen does not usually take part in the combustive reaction. Since it is important that there be enough oxygen for stochiometric combustion, and since air is cheap, combustion is usually accomplished with excess air.

Air Composition:

	Mass %	*Volume %*
O_2	23.2	21.0
N_2	76.8	79.0

Example

Expand the previous example of the combustion of octane to a reaction with 40% excess air by weight.

$$C_8H_{18} + 17.5O_2 + 66N_2 \longrightarrow 8CO_2 + 9H_2O + 5O_2 + 66N_2.$$

Note that the 66 moles of N_2 is derived from the volumetric ratio in air since molar coefficients are equal to volumetric coefficients:

$$\text{moles } N_2 = 17.5 \times \frac{79}{21} = 66.$$

PROBLEMS

1. A furnace burns a fuel-oil mixture completely. The products contain 18.7 moles of N_2 per mole of O_2. What is the percentage excess air by weight?

   a. 20%.
   b. 25%.
   c. 18%.
   d. 40%.
   e. 6%.

2. There are 11.3 moles of CO_2 per mole of fuel and 13.4 moles H_2O per mole of fuel. What is the percentage of carbon in the fuel?

   a. 66%.
   b. 16%.
   c. 76%.
   d. 84%.
   e. 54%.

Check your answers.

Answers

1. b.
2. d.

D. AFTERNOON PROBLEM SET

The following problem set is typical of the type of problem encountered in the afternoon section of the Engineering Fundamentals Examination. You will be expected to work five such problems in four hours.

COMBUSTION

Methane, CH_4, is burned in air completely.

1. Assuming stoichiometric ratios, how many moles of nitrogen are there in the products per lb of fuel?

   a. 7.5. b. 6.7. c. 5.2. d. 8.7. e. 2.

2. How many cubic feet of air must be provided per cubic feet of fuel, assuming they are at the same temperature?

   a. 10. b. 8.7. c. 9.5. d. 11.5. e. 5.7.

3. If outdoor air at 0°F is provided and the methane is supplied at 70°F, what is the volumetric fuel/air ratio?

   a. 9.5. b. 8.3. c. 0.12. d. 0.46. e. 0.57.

4. The process is changed to 20% excess air. lb O_2/lb fuel in the products = ?

   a. 2.0. b. 32. c. 4.8. d. 0.4. e. 0.8.

5. A volumetric analysis of the dry products above yields what percentage of CO_2?

   a. 8.1. b. 9.6. c. 10.2. d. 11.0. e. 13.2.

6. The analysis above is called:

   a. Redox. b. Orsat. c. Mollier. d. Molal. e. Avogadro.

7. How many lb of O_2 would you supply per lb of fuel to yield the maximum amount of carbon black in the products?

   a. 4. b. 3. c. 2. d. 1. e. 0.5.

8. In this reaction, what is the difference between the high-heat value and low-heat value for methane?

   a. 1050. b. 897. c. 1164. d. 952. e. 2360.

9. The fuel is changed to a mixture C_xH_y. With stoichiometric combustion a dry flue gas analysis shows 15% CO_2 by volume. What is the %C in the fuel by weight?

   a. 85. b. 25. c. 20. d. 66. e. 75.

10. The molecular weight of the fuel C_xH_y is:

    a. 380. b. 260. c. 210. d. 510. e. 240.

Check your answers.

Answers

1. a.
2. c.
3. c.
4. e.
5. b.
6. b.
7. c.
8. e.
9. a.
10. c.

11 Thermodynamics

Discussion of and problems related to the First Law of Thermodynamics, specific heat, the open system, the Second Law of Thermodynamics, equations of state, the Perfect Gas Law as an equation of state, equations of state for real gases, equations of state for two-phase fluids, and vapor cycles.

A. INTRODUCTION

Thermodynamics, as its name implies, deals with the movement or transfer of energy. The vehicle for energy transfer is either heat, work, or mass. The basic thermodynamic model is the *system* defined in such a way that heat, work, or mass crosses the system boundary at a steady rate. The working medium in thermodynamics is usually a fluid, a liquid, or, more often, a gas. For example, in the simple system below, the dotted line represents the system boundary. Heat, represented by Q, crosses the boundary from the flame to the water.

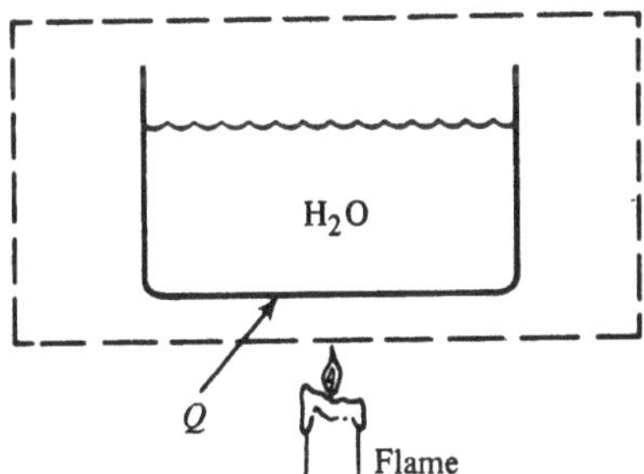

The *state* of a system describes its condition at a point in time. In the example above, state 1 could be the time when the flame was ignited, and state 2 could be one hour later.

The condition of a system at a given state is defined by *properties*. In the example, the temperature of the water is the relevant property state that describes the system. In other systems pressure and volume may be relevant properties. Temperature, pressure, and volume are the measurable properties. Thermodynamics also deals with other inferred properties which are not directly measurable. These will be covered later.

Heat flow, work flow, and mass flow are *not* properties. They are path variables which describe the means of getting from one state to another. But, since there are many paths possible between states, the properties do *not* depend on the path variables.

- Heat, work, or mass crosses the system boundaries.
- The state of the system is its condition at a point in time.
- Pressure, temperature, and volume are properties.
- Heat and work are path variables.

Example

Consider the previous container of water being heated by a flame:

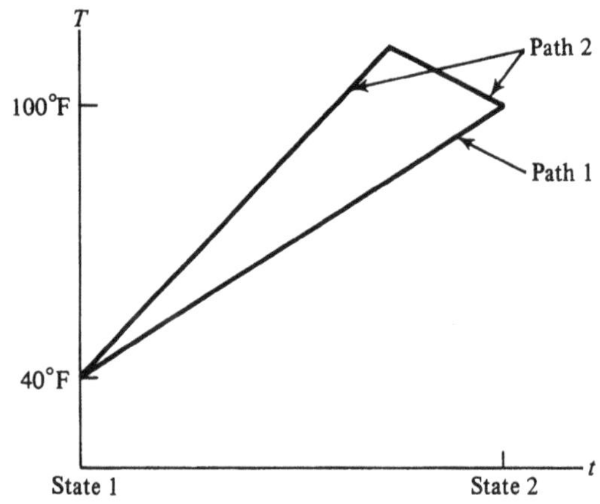

Path 1 represents a steady flame. Path 2 represents a larger flame which heats the water to a higher temperature but is turned off before the time associated with state 2 is reached. In both cases the properties of state 1 and state 2 are represented by 40°F and 100°F, respectively.

PROBLEMS

1. The condition of a thermodynamic system at a point in time is defined by:

   a. Its state.
   b. Temperature and pressure.
   c. Properties.
   d. The thermodynamic process.
   e. Work applied.

2. The measurable properties of a thermodynamic system can be related by:

   a. Avogadro's Law.
   b. The Helmholtz Function.
   c. The Maxwell Equations.
   d. The Ideal Gas Law.
   e. The Gibbs Function.

Check your answers.

Answers

1. c.
2. d.
   If you had difficulty with this problem, refer to Chapter 9.

B. THE FIRST LAW OF THERMODYNAMICS

The First Law of Thermodynamics is an energy-conservation law. The Second Law of Thermodynamics, which will be discussed later, states that most thermodynamic processes do not permit a balance between energy flowing into a system and energy flowing out. Conservation of energy, then, requires that any difference between inflow and outflow must be stored in the system.

Consider a cylinder and piston designed so that internal pressure is constant:

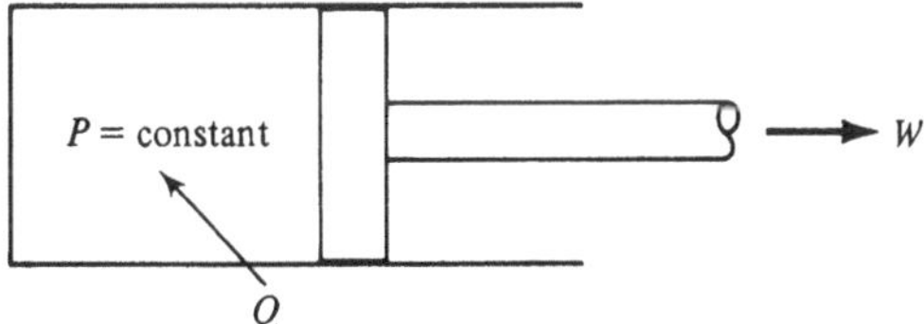

In this case, $Q - W = \Delta U$, where ΔU is the internal energy stored in the system. The above equation is the general statement of the First Law of Thermodynamics. The sign convention is that positive heat flows into the system and positive work flows out of the system. The symbol convention is that upper-case letters mean energy in Btu. Lower-case letters are called specific quantities in Btu/lb of fluid.

Internal energy is a thermodynamic property representing energy stored within a system. Two potentials can cause energy to move: (1) temperature causes heat to flow, and (2) pressure causes work to flow. In the constant-pressure process described, no change occurs in the pressure potential; therefore internal energy is a function of temperature alone.

A similar property combining the pressure and temperature potential is called *enthalpy*, represented by the letter H:

$$\Delta H = \Delta U + \Delta(pV).$$

The First Law of Thermodynamics in terms of enthalpy is:

$$Q - W = \Delta H - \Delta(pV).$$

Note that the pV term has the units of ft-lb (work). To convert it to Btu, use 778 ft-lb/Btu.

A closed thermodynamic process is one in which no mass is transferred across the system boundary. Four important processes to consider are listed below.

1. The Constant-Pressure (Isobaric) System

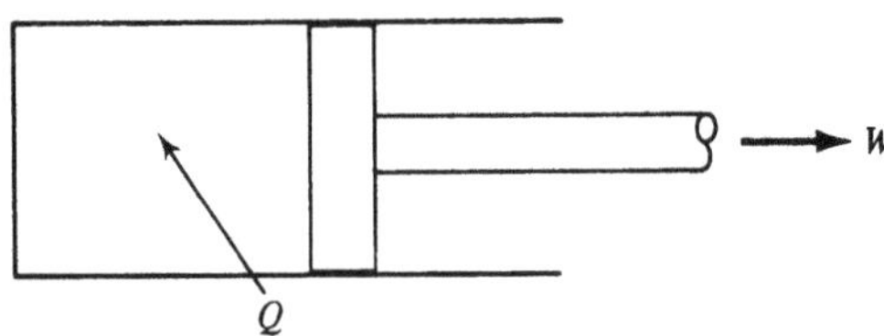

$$\Delta H = \Delta U + p\,\Delta V.$$

But since $W = \int_1^2 p\,dV$,

$$\Delta H = \Delta U + W.$$

Or, from the equation for the First Law,

$$\Delta H = Q.$$

2. The Constant-Volume (Isometric) System

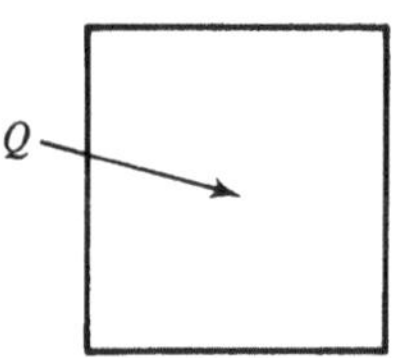

$$\Delta U = Q - W \qquad \text{(but } W = 0\text{)}.$$

So $\Delta U = Q$. But since $\Delta H = \Delta U + \Delta(pV)$,

$$\Delta H - V\,dp = Q.$$

3. The Constant-Temperature (Isothermal) System

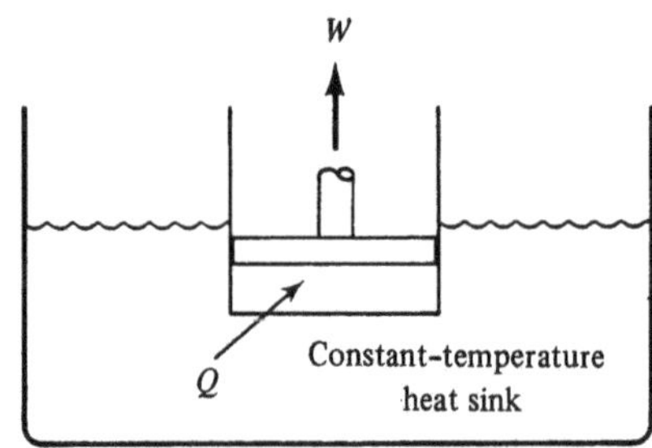

$$\Delta U = 0$$

$$\Delta H = \Delta(pV)$$

$$Q = W.$$

Note: A process such as this is called reversible because if the energy flows were reversed, $Q = W$ still holds.

4. The Adiabatic Process (No Heat Flow)

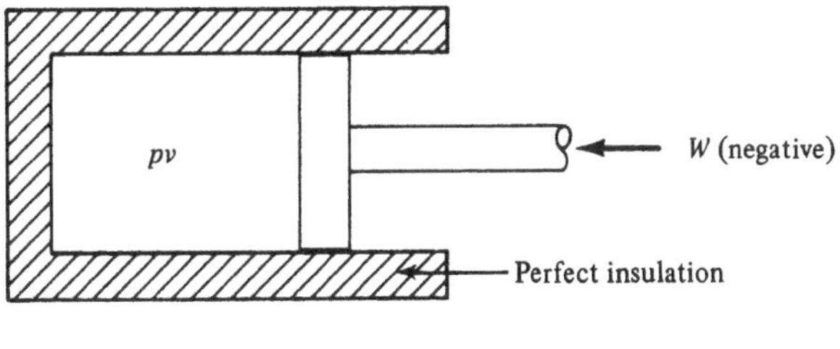

$$\Delta U = Q - W \qquad (Q = 0).$$

Therefore,

$$\Delta U = -W.$$

Note that if this process is carried out slowly and without friction, it is reversible. A reversible adiabatic process is called an *isentropic process.*

First Thermodynamic Law–Summary	
Isobaric process	$Q = \Delta H$
Isometric process	$Q = \Delta U$
Isothermal process	$Q = W$
Adiabatic process	$\Delta U = -W$

Example

A piston engine undergoes an enthalpy reduction of 5 Btu of its working fluid in each work-producing stroke. Assume this is adiabatic expansion due to the rapid movement of the piston and the fact that heat flow is a function of time. What is the work produced due to this expansion?

For the adiabatic process, $\Delta U = -W$. But, since

$$\Delta H = \Delta U + p\,\Delta V + V\,\Delta p$$

$$\Delta H = -W + p\,\Delta V + V\,\Delta p;$$

work due to volume change is $p\,\Delta V$. Therefore,

$\Delta H = V\,\Delta p$ equals work due to pressure drop;

$$\Delta H = W,$$

$$W = (5)(778) = 3890 \text{ ft-lb}.$$

PROBLEMS

1. In a constant-pressure system, work of 50 Btu is done on the system. Heat of 20 Btu is removed from the system. What is the change in internal energy?

   a. + 70 Btu.
   b. - 30 Btu.
   c. + 30 Btu.
   d. - 70 Btu.
   e. + 20 Btu.

2. A gasoline engine develops 50 horsepower and is 25% efficient. The heat rejection from the radiator is nearest to:

   a. 200 Btu/s.
   b. 140 Btu/s.
   c. 35 Btu/s.
   d. 70 Btu/s.
   e. 180 Btu/s.

Check your answers.

Answers

1. c.
2. b.

C. SPECIFIC HEAT

The heat capacity of a material is a function of temperature:

$$Q = C\,\Delta T.$$

Specific heat refers to the heat capacity of a unit mass of the material:

$$Q = mc\,\Delta T$$

or

$$q = c\,\Delta T.$$

For example, the specific heat of water is 1 Btu/lb-°F, which is the definition of Btu.

When dealing with gases, it is necessary to define two specific heats, one at constant pressure and one at constant volume. These specific heats are properties of the fluid and can be found in a handbook of such properties.

Constant Pressure:

$$Q = mc_p \, \Delta T = \Delta H.$$

Constant Volume:

$$Q = mc_V \, \Delta T = \Delta U.$$

Ideal Gas:

$$c_p - c_V = \frac{R}{\text{mw}} = \frac{1546}{(\text{mw})(J)} = \frac{1.99}{\text{mw}}.$$

where
m = mass in lb_m of the gas
mw = molecular weight of the gas
J = 778 lb-ft/Btu

Example

What is the enthalpy change for a pound of ideal gas that has a ratio

$$K = \frac{c_p}{c_V} = 1.4$$

and a gas constant of 53.3, if the temperature is increased by 200°F?

$$c_p = \left(\frac{R}{J}\right)\left(\frac{K}{K-1}\right) = \frac{(53.3)(1.4)}{(778)(0.4)} = 0.24 \text{ Btu/lb-°F}$$

$$\Delta h = c_p \, \Delta T = (0.24)(200) = 48 \text{ Btu/lb}.$$

PROBLEMS

1. In the previous example, the numbers used are those for air. If 20 Btu of work is done on 1 lb of air in the process, what is the heat flow?

   a. + 54 Btu/lb.
   b. + 14 Btu/lb.
   c. - 14 Btu/lb.
   d. + 28 Btu/lb.
   e. - 28 Btu/lb.

2. The following data are for a gas at low pressures. (The ideal gas law does *not* apply.)

T (°R)	u (Btu/lb)
200	33.96
220	37.38
240	40.80

What is specific heat at constant volume?

a. 1.4.
b. 1.7.
c. 0.24.
d. 0.17.
e. 2.4.

Check your answers.

Answers

1. d.
   $c_V = 0.17$. Check sign convention for W and Q.
2. d.

D. THE OPEN SYSTEM

Real processes often rely on the flow of working fluids. To consider any element in a process as a thermodynamic system, we must consider a system where mass crosses the system boundary. This requires a different definition of the state of a system. Rather than at a point in time, consider the state of a given pound of the fluid flowing at some rate through the system. This can be illustrated as follows:

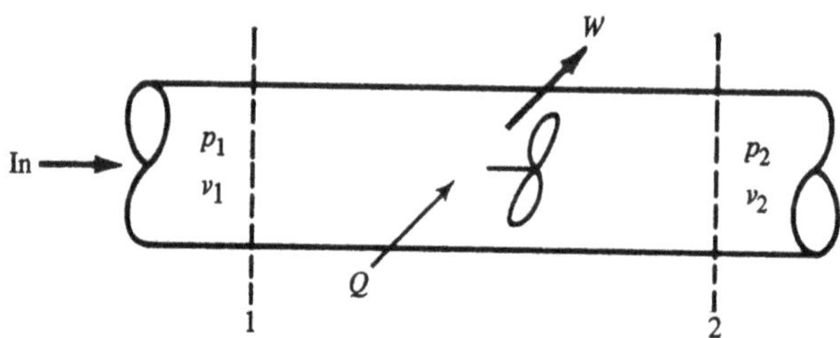

The equation for the First Law becomes:

$$q - w = \Delta u + \frac{\Delta(pV)}{J} + \frac{\Delta(\dot{x}^2)}{2gJ}$$

or

$$q - w = \Delta h + \frac{\Delta \dot{x}^2}{2gJ}.$$

where $\dot{x} = \dfrac{dx}{dt}$ (velocity)

Example

Consider the gas flow in the following pipe:

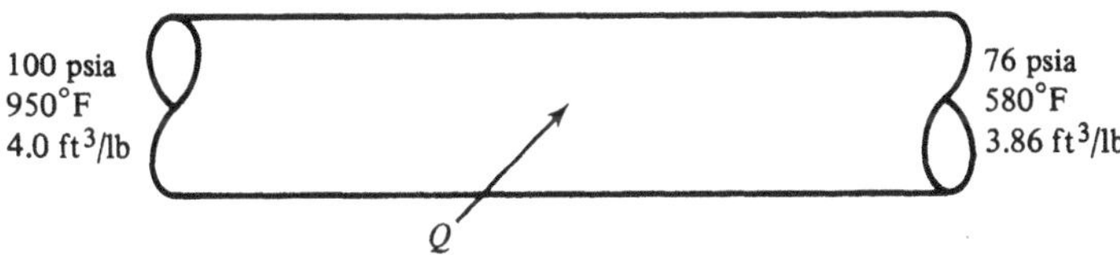

Given $c_V = 0.32$, what is Q?

$$q - w = \Delta u + \Delta \frac{pv}{J} + \frac{(\dot{x}^2)}{2g}$$

$$W = 0.$$

Assume $\dot{x}$ is negligible.

$$q = \Delta u + \Delta \frac{pv}{J}$$

$$= u_2 - u_1 + p_2 v_2 - p_1 v_1$$

$$= c_V (T_2 - T_1) + p_2 v_2 - p_1 v_1$$

$$= 0.32[(580 + 460) - (950 + 460)] + \frac{(76)(144)(3.86)}{778} - \frac{(100)(144)(4)}{778}$$

$$= -138.2 \text{ Btu/lb}.$$

The minus sign means heat is removed from the system.

PROBLEMS

1. An adiabatic steam turbine receives steam at state 1 and rejects steam at state 2:

$$h_1 = 1400 \text{ Btu/lb}, \qquad h_2 = 1200 \text{ Btu/lb},$$

$$\dot{x}_1 = 110 \text{ ft/s}, \qquad \dot{x}_2 = 810 \text{ ft/s}.$$

How much work does the turbine do?

a. 213 Btu/lb.
b. 225 Btu/lb.
c. 183 Btu/lb.
d. 164 Btu/lb.
e. 280 Btu/lb.

2. Which of the following processes will result in compression of a gas with the least work input?

a. Polytropic.
b. Isothermal.
c. Adiabatic.
d. Isobaric.
e. Isometric.

Check your answers.

Answers

1. c.
2. b.

E. THE SECOND LAW OF THERMODYNAMICS

Work can be produced continuously only if a work-producing process is followed by a process which returns the system to its initial conditions. Consider the constant temperature process below.

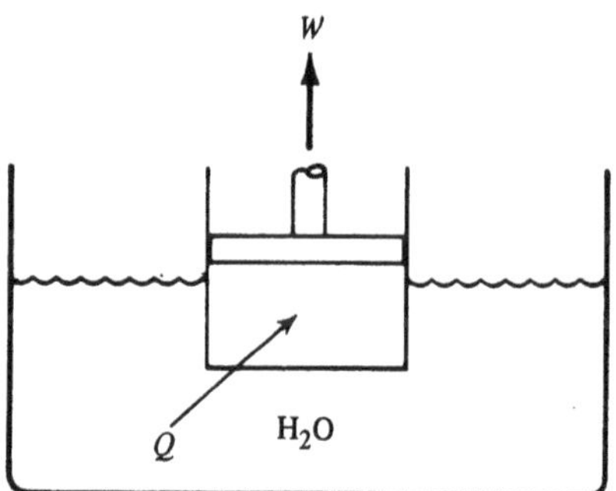

To return the piston to its initial position to complete a cycle would consume as much work as was produced. To overcome this difficulty, the temperature of the water can be reduced to cause heat to flow out of the system. The amount of work lost in returning to initial conditions is proportional to this lower temperature.

The result is that heat cannot be continuously converted to work with 100% efficiency because a cycle cannot consist totally of reversible processes.

The ideal cycle for converting heat to work is the *Carnot cycle* plotted on a pV diagram below:

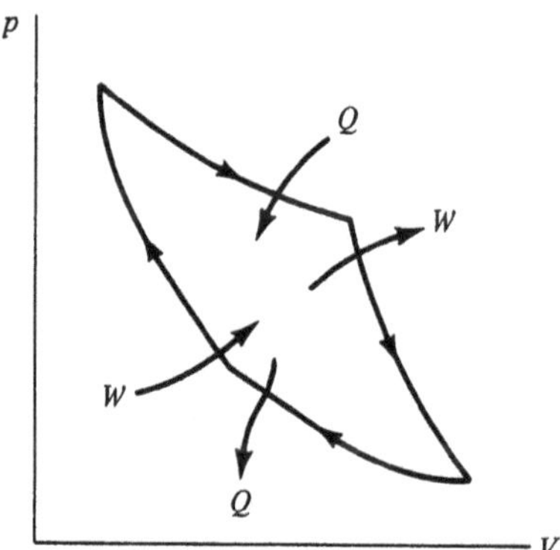

Efficiency is

$$\eta = \frac{Q_{in} - Q_{out}}{Q_{in}} = 1 - \frac{Q_{out}}{Q_{in}}$$

Since $Q \propto T$,

$$\eta = 1 - \frac{T_{out}}{T_{in}}.$$

The Carnot efficiency represents the highest possible efficiency for a cycle operating between two temperatures and obviously cannot equal 100% unless T_{out} is 0°R.

The lack of reversibility in a cycle of thermodynamic processes is proportional to a property called *entropy*. Entropy is a property which is constant during any adiabatic process. In a nonadiabatic process, entropy decreases if heat leaves the system and increases if heat is added to the system. In the Carnot cycle mentioned previously, more heat enters on expansion than leaves on compression. Hence the cycle results in a net increase in entropy. This is a measure of cycle irreversibility.

> Entropy is represented as a function of the temperature and pressure of the substance. In the English system, the unit of entropy is Btu/lb-°R.
>
> Algebraically:
>
> $$\Delta S = \int \frac{dQ_{rev}}{T}$$
>
> or
>
> $$T\,dS = dU + p\,dV$$
>
> $$T\,dS = dH + V\,dp.$$

Example

If we wished to find the change in entropy associated with boiling 1 lb of water at 200 psia:

From the steam tables, $T = 381.8$°F.

Heat of vaporization = 843 Btu/lb.

Since this is a reversible isothermal process,

$$\Delta S = \frac{Q}{T} = \frac{843}{381.8 + 460} = 1.002 \text{ Btu/lb-°R}.$$

For the case where T is not constant,

$$s_2 - s_1 = \int_1^2 \frac{dq_{rev}}{T} = \int_1^2 \frac{c\,dT}{T}$$

$$= c \ln(T_2/T_1).$$

This will describe the change in entropy between points 1 and 2 achieved by any process, reversible or not.

PROBLEMS

1. In the Carnot cycle efficiency depends primarily on:

   a. Lack of friction.
   b. Adiabatic expansion.
   c. A low-temperature heat sink.
   d. A high temperature difference.
   e. Reversible processes.

2. In a constant-pressure process $\Delta S = \frac{1}{2}c_p$. If the initial temperature is 200°F, what is the final temperature?

   a. 635°F.
   b. 330°F.
   c. 398°F.
   d. 120°F.
   e. 730°F.

Check your answers.

Answers

1. d.
2. a.
   Use the definition in the example; temperatures are in °R.

F. EQUATIONS OF STATE

An equation of state is a functional relationship between the properties of one state and another. Basically two basic types of equations of state exist:

Equations of State:
1. Perfect Gas Laws;
2. Gas Tables for Real Fluids.

Example

The perfect gas law as an equation of state:

$$pV = nRT, \qquad R = 1545.3 \frac{\text{ft-lb}}{\text{lb-mole-}^\circ\text{R}}$$

$$n = \frac{\text{mass}}{\text{molecular weight}}.$$

For example, how much nitrogen gas is there in a container of 120 in^3 at 73°F and 200 psig?

$$(200 + 14.7)(144)\frac{(120)}{(1728)} = m\frac{(1545)}{(28)}(460 + 73)$$

$$m = 0.073 \text{ lb.}$$

PROBLEM

Which of the following is *not* an equation of state?

a. The Ideal Gas Law.
b. Van der Waal's Equation.
c. The slope on a pV diagram.
d. Keenan and Keyes Tables.
e. The Mollier Diagram.

Check your answer.

Answer

c.
Use a dictionary or the index in your thermodynamics text for definitions.

G. THE PERFECT GAS LAW AS AN EQUATION OF STATE

In a previous chapter (Chapter 9), the Perfect Gas Law was used for relating the measurable properties pV and T for two states. The inferred properties, U, H, and S can also be so related as the following table indicates. Table 3 lists the equations of state for the four thermody-

TABLE 3. Equations of State

Process	Constant-volume (isometric)	Constant-pressure (isobaric)	Constant-temperature (isothermal)	Reversible adiabatic (isentropic) $pV^k = C$	Polytropic $pV^n = c$
p-V-T relations	$\frac{T_2}{T_1} = \frac{p_2}{p_1}$	$\frac{T_2}{T_1} = \frac{V_2}{V_1}$	$p_1V_1 = p_2V_2$	$p_1V^k = p_2V_2^k$	$p_1V_1^n = p_2V_2^n$
$W = \int p\,dV$	0	$p(V_2 - V_1)$	$p_1V_1 \ln\frac{V_2}{V_1}$	$\frac{p_2V_2 - p_1V_1}{1 - k}$	$\frac{p_2V_2 - p_1V_1}{1 - n}$
$U_2 - U_1$	$mc_V(T_2 - T_1)$	$mc_V(T_2 - T_1)$	0	$mc_V(T_2 - T_1)$	$mc_V(T_2 - T_1)$
$H_2 - H_1$	$mc_p(T_2 - T_1)$	$mc_p(T_2 - T_1)$	0	$mc_p(T_2 - T_1)$	$mc_p(T_2 - T_1)$
$S_2 - S_1$	$mc_V \ln\frac{T_2}{T_1}$	$mc_p \ln\frac{T_2}{T_1}$	$\frac{mR}{J}\ln\frac{V_2}{V_1}$	0	$mc_n \ln\frac{T_2}{T_1}$

NOTE: $K = C_p/C_v$ in the isentropic process.

namic properties discussed so far and for one other—the *polytropic process.* A polytropic process is any process which is not one of the first four: isometric, isobaric, isothermal, or adiabatic.

Example

In a polytropic process we make use of the fact that the properties of a state do not depend on the path between them. In the process A–B shown below,

- p is not constant,
- V is not constant,
- T is not constant, and
- S is not constant,

meaning the process is *not* adiabatic.

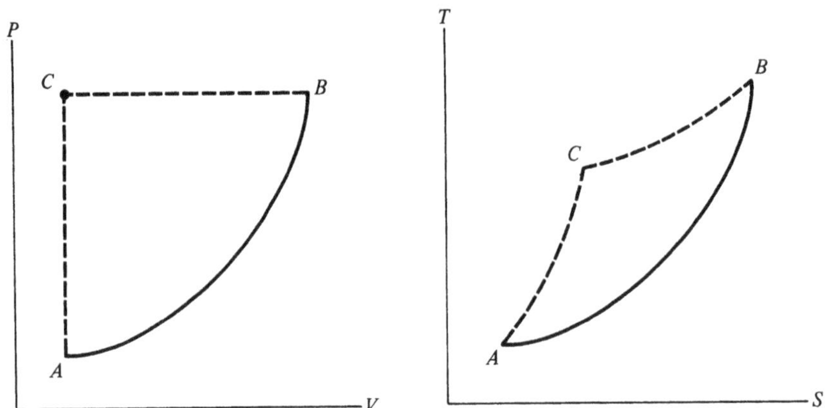

Look at the constant-volume process A–C and the constant-pressure process C–B. Together these will have the same end states as A–B:

$$\Delta S = \int_A^B \frac{dQ}{T} = \int_A^C \frac{c_V \, \Delta T}{T}\bigg|_V + \int_C^B \frac{c_p \, \Delta T}{T}\bigg|_p$$

$$= c_V \ln \frac{T_C}{T_A}\bigg|_V + c_p \ln \frac{T_B}{T_C}\bigg|_p .$$

From the Perfect Gas Law,

$$\frac{T_C}{T_A} = \frac{p_C}{p_A} = \frac{p_B}{p_A} \quad \text{and} \quad \frac{T_B}{T_C} = \frac{V_B}{V_C} = \frac{V_B}{V_A} .$$

Therefore,

$$\Delta S = c_V \ln \frac{p_B}{p_A} + c_p \ln \frac{V_B}{V_A} .$$

PROBLEMS

1. In a Carnot engine:

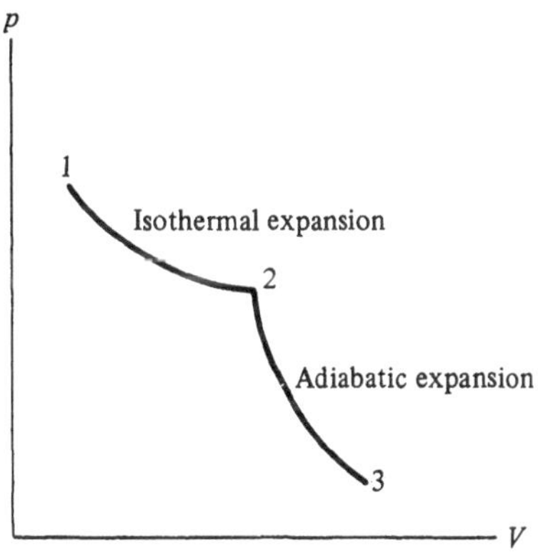

$$p_1 = 60 \text{ psia}$$
$$V_1 = 2 \text{ ft}^3$$
$$p_3 = 10 \text{ psia}$$
$$V_3 = 7 \text{ ft}^3.$$

The efficiency is:

a. 58%.
b. 64%.
c. 38%.
d. 50%.
e. 42%.

2. In the constant-pressure process with air from 100°F to 50°F, the specific entropy change is:

a. - 0.166 Btu/lb-°F.
b. + 0.166 Btu/lb-°F.
c. - 0.022 Btu/lb-°F.
d. + 0.022 Btu/lb-°F.
e. None of the above.

Check your answers.

Answers

1. e.
   Refer to section E for the efficiency of a Carnot engine.
2. c.

H. EQUATIONS OF STATE FOR REAL GASES

The equivalent of the Perfect Gas Law for real gases is a set of gas tables which tabulate the properties over a range of values.

> Gas tables are the equivalent of the Perfect Gas Law for real gases.

Example

The properties of air at low pressure are as follows for the two temperatures indicated. (NOTE: You should have more extensive tables from a good text in thermodynamics with you for the examination.)

T (°R)	h (Btu/lb)	u (Btu/lb)	s (Btu/lb-°R)
530	126	90	0.596
860	206	147	0.713

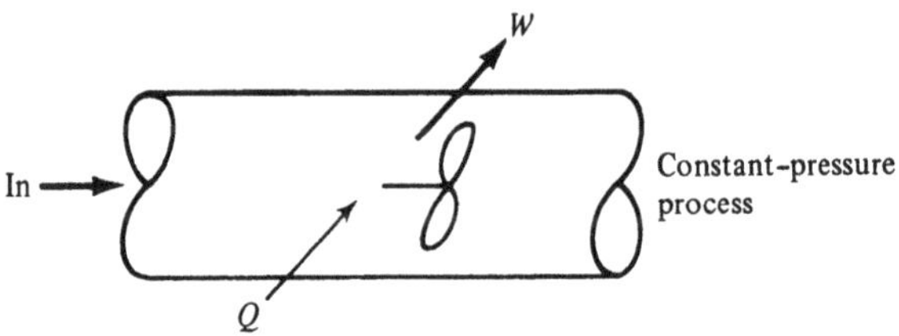

$$q = h_2 - h_1 = 206 - 126 = 80 \text{ Btu/lb}$$

$$\Delta s = 0.713 - 0.596 = 0.1169 \text{ Btu/lb-°R}$$

$$w = p\,\Delta v = \Delta h - \Delta u$$

$$= 80 - (147 - 90) = 23 \text{ Btu/lb.}$$

PROBLEM

The molecular weight of air is 29. What is the error in heat flow in the example above if air is considered to be a perfect gas?

a. 0.8 Btu/lb.
b. 1.0 Btu/lb.
c. 4.4 Btu/lb.
d. 0.04 Btu/lb.
e. 1.2 Btu/lb.

Check your answer.

Answer

a.

I. EQUATIONS OF STATE FOR TWO-PHASE FLUIDS

Thermodynamic systems often use gaseous and liquid phases of the same fluid in equilibrium. The steam engine and refrigeration machines are two common examples. The following discussion will use steam as an example, although the principles apply to any gas/liquid system.

The *TS* diagram is most often used to illustrate the two-phase system with a vapor dome separating the phases:

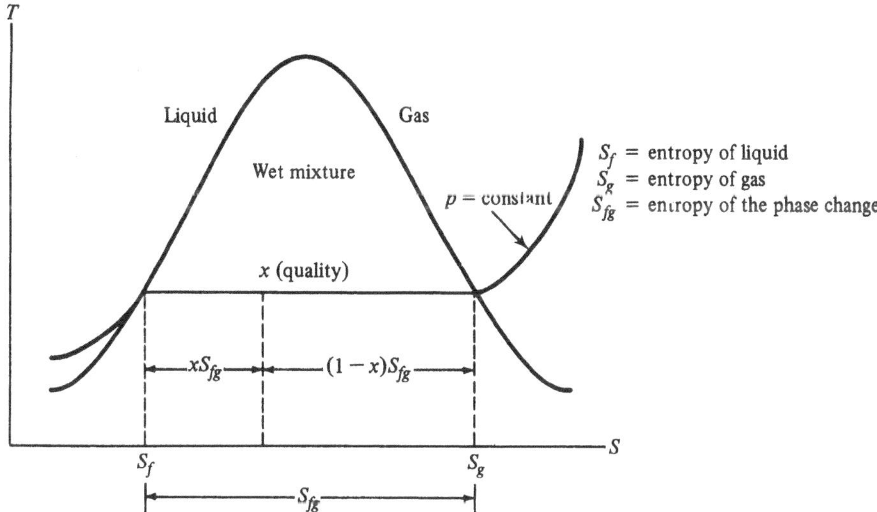

x is the quality of the saturated mixture; $(1 - x)$ is the moisture content. Steam tables are available listing all the thermodynamic properties for saturated steam and for superheated steam. Also, an h–s diagram called a Mollier Chart is available.

For analysis of the properties in the regions delineated above, use the following rules:

Liquid Region (subcooled liquid):
- Use specific heat of liquid.

Wet-Mixture Region (saturated liquid):
- Use saturated steam tables and the following relationships:

$$h = h_f + xh_{fg}$$

$$s = s_f + xs_{fg}.$$

Gas Region (superheated steam):
- Use superheated steam tables or a Mollier Diagram.

Example

Saturated steam is superheated in a boiler at constant pressure. Determine the final state if the initial pressure is 500 psia and a final condition in which the steam has 200°F superheat is desired. How much energy per pound of fluid is added to superheat the steam?

A Mollier Diagram for this process is shown below:

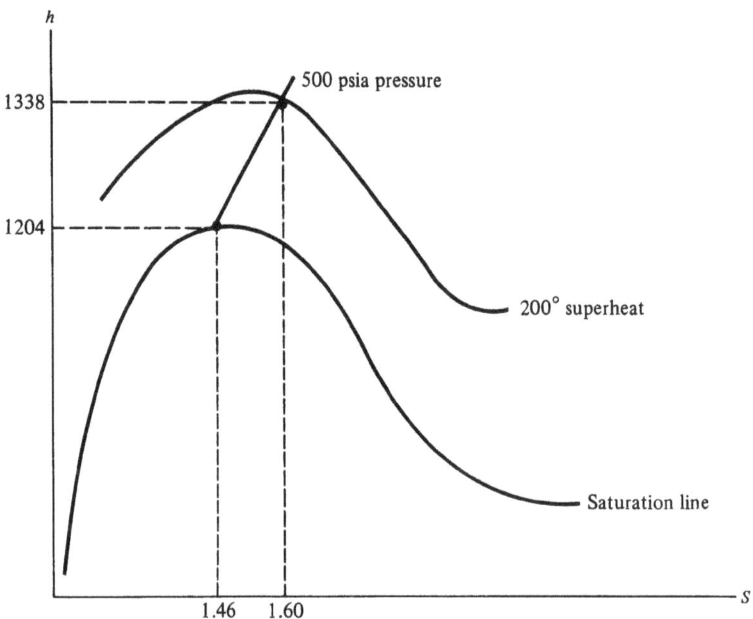

Proceeding from the saturation line at 500 psia to a line of 200°F superheat yields h = 1338 Btu/lb and s = 1.60 Btu/lb-°R. For saturation, h = 1204.4 Btu/lb. Since the process is a steady-flow process at constant pressure, the energy equation becomes $q = h_2 - h_1$ if differences in kinetic-energy and potential-energy terms are negligible. Therefore, q = 1338 - 1204.4 = 133.6 Btu/lb.

PROBLEMS

1. An isentropic steam turbine operates between state 1 and state 2:

State 1	*State 2*
h = 1525 Btu/lb	h = 1300 Btu/lb
$\dot{x}$ = 110 ft/sec	$\dot{x}$ = 810 ft/sec

Shaft work is:

a. 184 Btu/lb.
b. 212 Btu/lb.
c. 238 Btu/lb.
d. 616 Btu/lb.
e. 196 Btu/lb.

2. How much heat is extracted in a steam condenser if steam enters at 1 in. Hg and 15% moisture?

a. 974 Btu/lb.
b. 69.7 Btu/lb.
c. 1044 Btu/lb.
d. 892 Btu/lb.
e. 144 Btu/lb.

3. The boiling point of ammonia (NH_3) at 30 psia is 0°F and at 130 psia is 71°F. What is its state at 71°F and 140 psia?

   a. Subcooled liquid.
   b. Saturated vapor.
   c. Superheated vapor.
   d. Eutectic.
   e. Triple point.

Check your answers.

Answers

1. b.
2. d.
3. a.

J. VAPOR CYCLES

Engines commonly take in air and fuel and exhaust gases (products of combustion). An exception to this is the steam cycle. In all cases, the engine can be approximated by an assumption that the engine is a closed system with heat and work crossing the boundaries.

The Rankine Cycle (Steam Turbine)

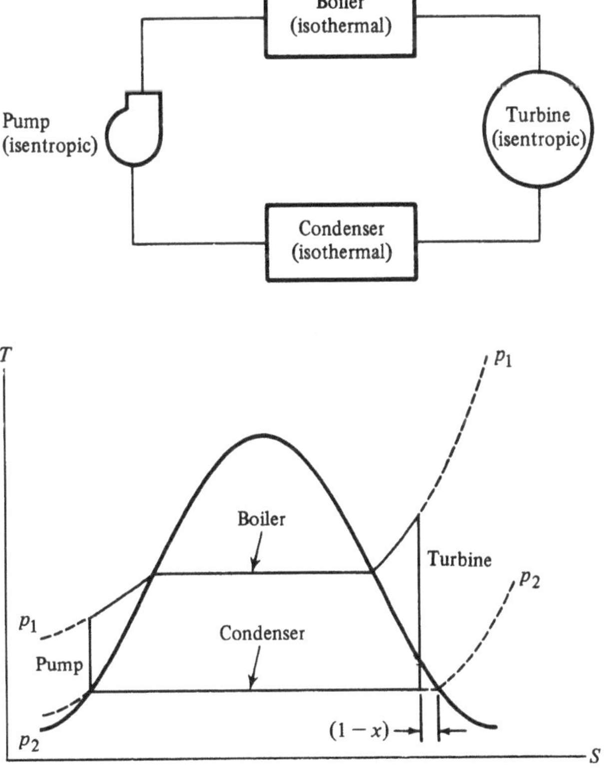

Since for an open isentropic system $w = \Delta h$,

$$\text{efficiency} = \frac{\Delta H_{\text{turbine}}}{\Delta H_{\text{turbine}} + \Delta H_{\text{condenser}}}.$$

NOTE: ΔH of the condenser is xh_{fg}.

The Reverse Vapor Cycle (Refrigeration)

The refrigeration cycle is very similar to the steam turbine. The refrigeration compressor is analogous to the turbine (isentropic), and the expansion valve is analogous to the pump except that it is isenthalpic (constant enthalpy) rather than isentropic.

Rankine Cycle:

$$w_{\text{pump}} = \Delta h$$
$$q_{\text{boiler}} = \Delta h$$
$$w_{\text{turbine}} = \Delta h$$
$$q_{\text{condenser}} = \Delta h.$$

Example

What is the work produced by the turbine shown below?

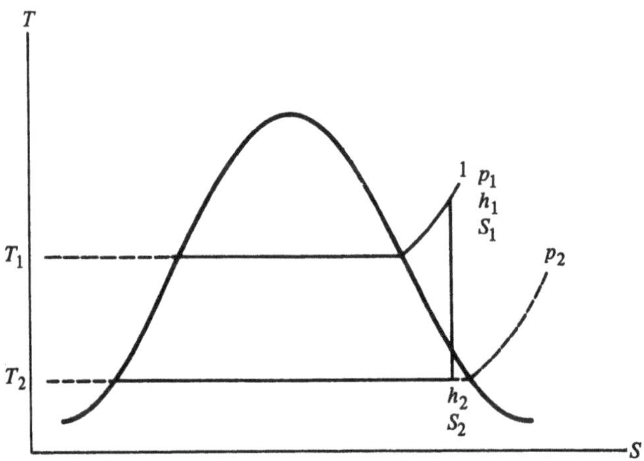

h_1 and s_1 can be read directly from superheated steam tables given T_1 and p_1. The quality at point 2 can be determined as follows:

$$s_1 = s_2 = s_f + xs_{fg}.$$

s_f and s_{fg} can be read from saturated tables given T_2 and p_2. Then knowing x (quality), enthalpy at point 2 is derived as follows:

$$h_2 = h_f + xh_{fg};$$

and work:

$$w = h_1 - h_2.$$

PROBLEM

A Rankine steam turbine operates from 600°F and 600 psia to an outlet of 1 psia. How much heat is removed from the condenser?

a. 1036 Btu/lb.
b. 1634 Btu/lb.
c. 786 Btu/lb.
d. 1978 Btu/lb.
e. 560 Btu/lb.

Check your answer.

Answer

c.
You will need steam tables for this problem.

K. AFTERNOON PROBLEM SET

The following problem set is typical of the type of problem encountered in the afternoon section of the Engineering Fundamentals Examination. You will be expected to work five such problems in four hours.

THERMODYNAMICS

The refrigeration system shown is operating with a refrigerant described in the table below between 5°F and 86°F.

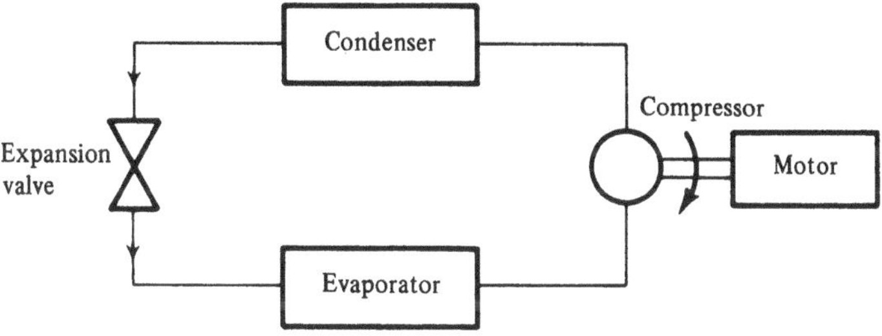

Refrigerant Table (Saturated Refrigerant)

Temperature (°F)	Pressure (psia)	Enthalpy			Entropy		
		h_f	h_{fg}	h_g	S_f	S_{fg}	S_g
5	25	6.7	68.2	74.9	0.015	0.155	0.170
75	90	24.1	63.4	87.6	0.048	0.120	0.168
86	110	27.2	59.5	86.7	0.055	0.110	0.165

Superheated Tables

Saturation pressure (psia)	Property	100°F	120°F	140°F	160°F
90	*h*	85.7	89.2	97.5	105.3
	S	0.166	0.168	0.186	0.192
110	*h*	88.2	92.4	98.3	101.2
	S	0.168	0.170	0.189	0.200
120	*h*		96.4	105.1	113.7
	S		0.180	0.194	0.206

1. Which of the following diagrams most closely describes the system?

a.

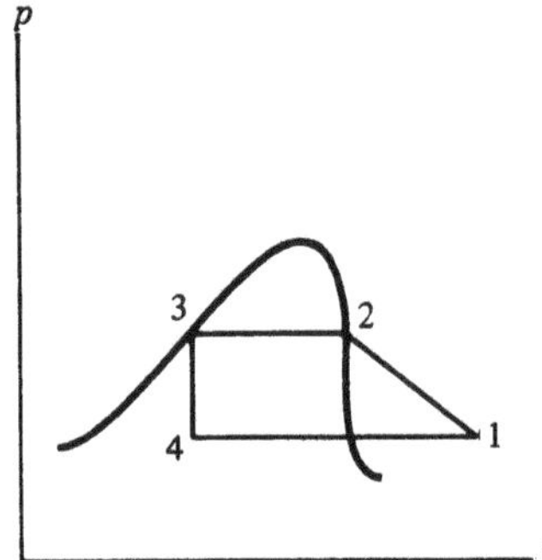

d.

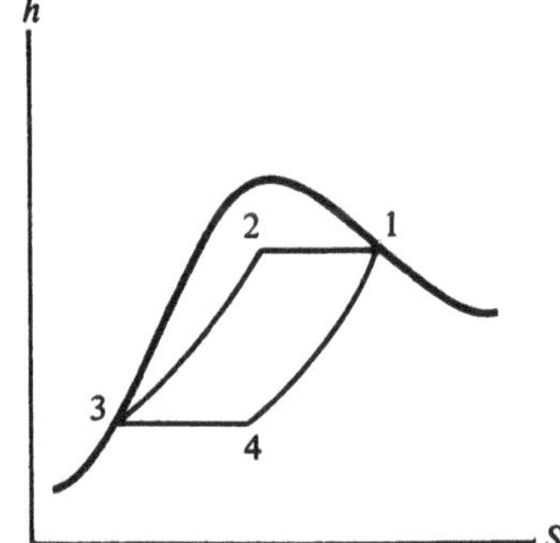

b.

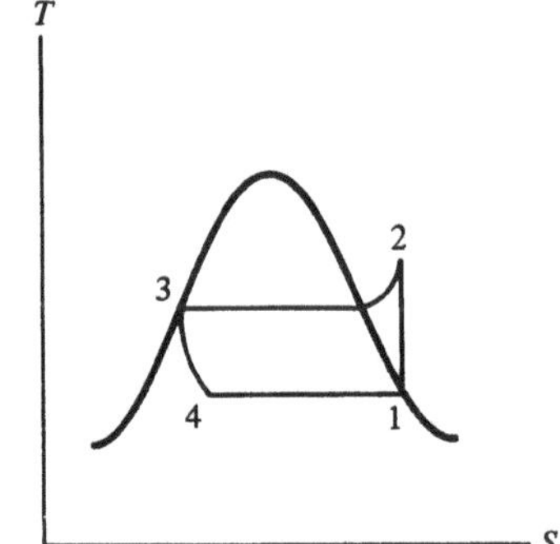

e.

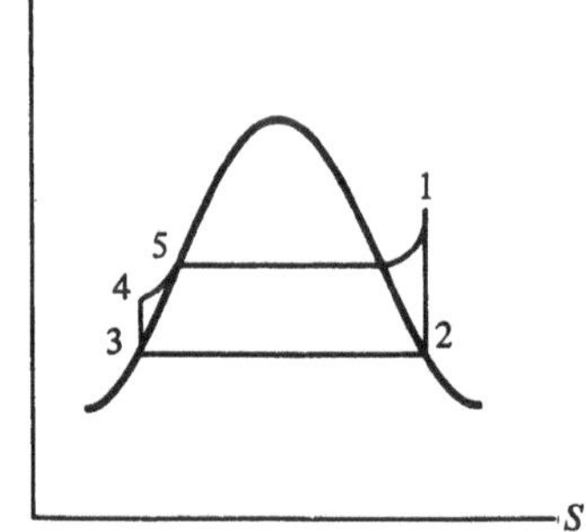

c.

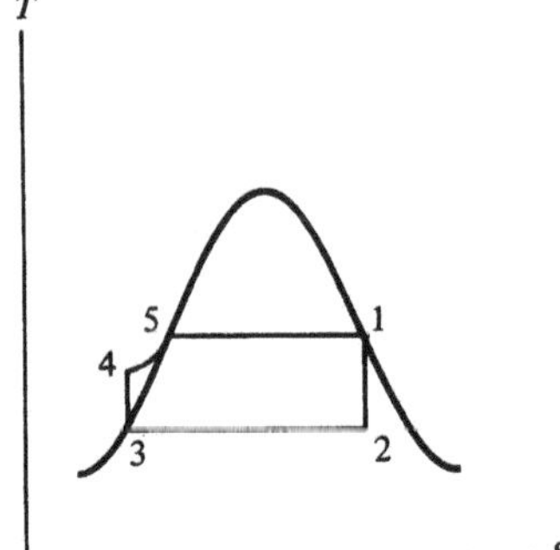

2. Which process represents compression?

   a. 1–2. c. 2–3. e. 1–3.
   b. 3–4. d. 4–1.

3. What is the temperature at the compressor outlet?

   a. 86°F. c. 100°F. e. 130°F.
   b. 92°F. d. 120°F.

4. How much heat in Btu/h is given up in the condenser if the mean flow rate is 240 lb/h?

   a. 17,800. c. 22,176. e. 15,648.
   b. 20,808. d. 14,280.

5. Suppose the condenser temperature is such that heat rejection totals 14,000 Btu/h. How many gpm of water would it take to produce a 10°F temperature rise across a water-cooled condenser?

   a. 1.4. c. 2.8. e. 5.0.
   b. 2.2. d. 4.8.

6. If the compressor has an efficiency of 85% of isentropic, what is the compressor outlet superheat?

   a. 62. c. 32. e. 14.
   b. 74. d. 84.

7. How much heat will be absorbed in the evaporator (Btu/lb)?

   a. 47.7. c. 59.5. e. 74.9.
   b. 68.2. d. 27.2.

8. If the mass-flow rate is 240 lb/h and the single-cylinder compressor has 3″ bore, 4″ stroke, what is the rpm if the compressor is isentropic, the volumetric efficiency is 100%, and the entering specific volume is 0.5 ft^3/lb?

   a. 645. c. 335. e. 122.
   b. 265. d. 42.

9. What is the Coefficient of Performance (COP)?

   a. 1.3. c. 3.2. e. 4.1.
   b. 2.7. d. 1.8.

10. Using the assumptions of Problem 8, what horsepower motor would you use?

    a. 0.5. c. 1.5. e. 2.5.
    b. 1.0. d. 2.0.

Check your answers.

Answers

1. b.
2. a.
3. d.
4. e.
5. c.
6. b.
7. a.
8. e.
9. b.
10. d.

12 Fluids

Discussion of and problems related to hydrostatics, buoyancy, fluid kinematics, fluid viscosity, friction energy, and hydrodynamics.

A. INTRODUCTION

By definition a fluid is a substance incapable of resisting a shearing force. This means that all forces transmitted by a fluid are normal to the surface of the fluid. Consider the fluid system below.

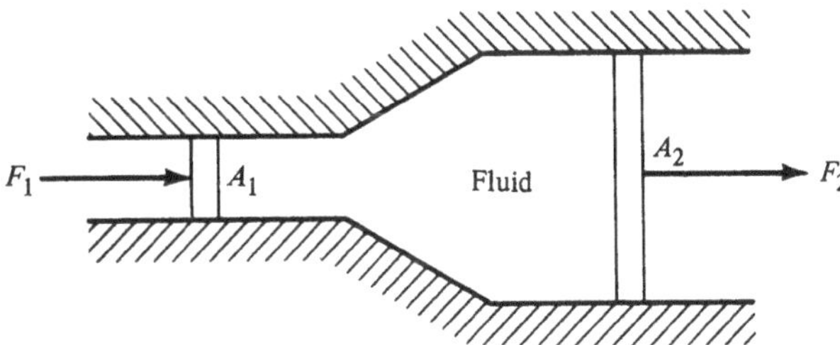

The force F_1 exerts a pressure $p = F_1/A_1$ on the fluid, which in turn exerts a force $F_2 = pA_2$ on the right-hand piston. In this static case, the pressure p is uniform and constant throughout the system. Accordingly, within the fluid system it becomes more meaningful to talk of pressure rather than forces.

Fluids fall into two categories, *compressible* and *incompressible*. Generally, compressible fluids are gases, while incompressible fluids are liquids. Specifically, gases have a density dependent on pressure and temperature (Perfect Gas Law), while liquids have a density that is independent of pressure and related to temperature only by its coefficient of thermal expansion. The primary emphasis in fluid mechanics is on incompressible fluids (liquids).

Incompressible Hydrostatic Fluids

In the absence of fluid flow, the governing functional relationship of a hydrostatic system is one of balancing forces or, in terms of pressure, constant pressure throughout the system.

Incompressible Kinematic Fluids

In cases of flowing fluids, friction and conservation of mass enter the functional relationship.

Hydraulic Systems

Historically systems involving the flow of water use a system of energy units based on "water head" in which all units are expressed in feet. For example, pressure-related potential energy, rather than being stated in terms of psi, is stated as the depth of the equivalent water column which will exert the subject pressure. The principal terms used in dealing with hydraulic systems are given in the table below, where w is density, v is velocity, and g is gravitational acceleration.

Pressure head	p/w
Potential energy head	Z
Kinetic velocity head	$v^2/2g$
Enthalpy	E

An energy conservation balance of these terms is called the *Bernoulli Equation.* It is analogous to the First Law of Thermodynamics.

Bernoulli Equation:

$$\Delta E + \frac{\Delta p}{w} + \Delta Z + \frac{\Delta v^2}{2g} = 0.$$

Example

A dam holds back 30 ft of water. What is the pressure on the gate of a closed valve at the bottom of the dam?

The only two energy terms in this example are gradient head (Z) and pressure head (p/w). Therefore,

$$\Delta p/w = \Delta Z$$

$$p = wZ = 62.4 \text{ lb/ft}^3 \times 30 \text{ ft}$$

$$= 1872 \text{ psf}$$

$$= 13 \text{ psi.}$$

PROBLEMS

1. If the valve in the previous example is opened, the velocity of water through it is nearest to:

   a. 32 ft/sec. c. 26 ft/sec. e. 64.4 ft/sec.
   b. 44 ft/sec. d. 52 ft/sec.

2. In the container shown below, the force on the stopper is:

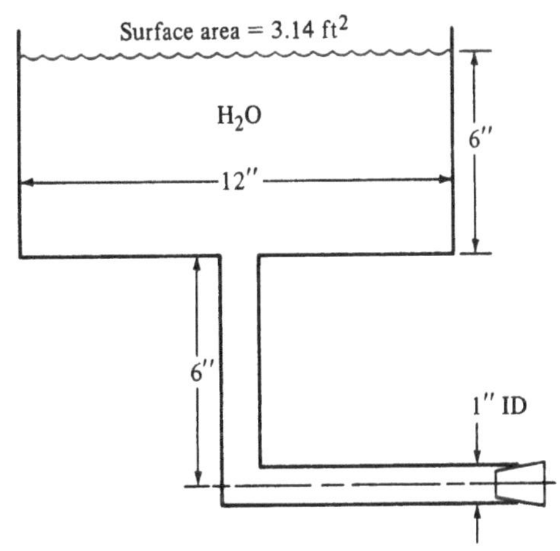

   a. 0.34 lb_f. c. 0.43 lb_f. e. 0.88 lb_f.
   b. 1.78 lb_f. d. 1.36 lb_f.

Check your answers.

Answers

1. b.
   $v = \sqrt{2gh}$.
2. a.

B. HYDROSTATICS

In the hydrostatics problem there are only gradient and pressure heads. The *manometer*, an important instrument for reading pressure, is a device for translating pressure head to gradient head.

Manometer

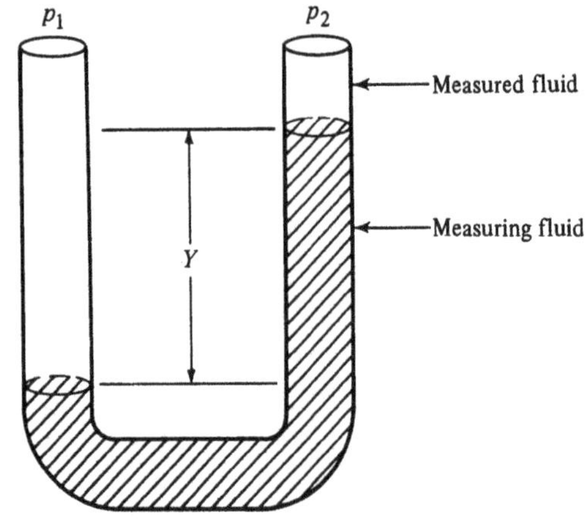

$$\frac{p_1}{w} - \frac{p_2}{w} = (1 - S)y.$$

$$S = \frac{w(\text{measured fluid})}{w(\text{measuring fluid})}.$$

p = pressure, lb/ft^2;
w = density, lb/ft^3 of measuring fluid;
S = specific gravity of measured fluid if w is density of H_2O.

NOTE: When air is used with water or mercury, S can be considered negligible.

Hydrostatic Forces on Plane Areas

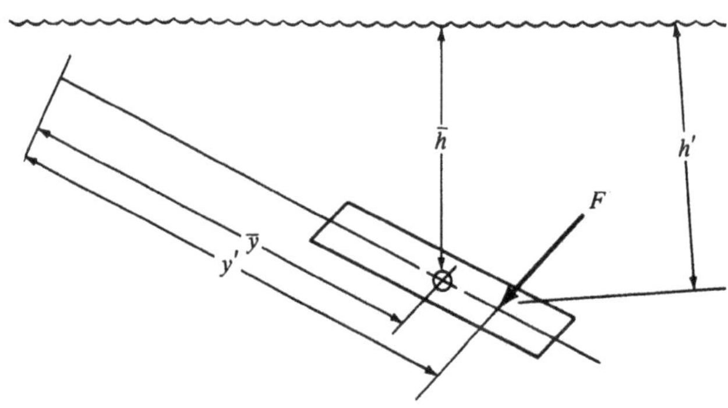

Equivalent Force:

$F = w \sin\theta \int y \, dA$

$= w \sin\theta \, \bar{y}A$

$F = w\bar{h}A.$

Center of Pressure (point of application):

$$y' = \bar{y} + \frac{I_g}{\bar{y}A},$$

where I_g is the area moment of inertia about the center of gravity, expressed in ft^4. Refer to Chapter 6 for a discussion of moment of inertia.

Hydrostatic Force:	
magnitude:	$F = w\bar{h}A;$
point of application:	$y' = \bar{y} + \frac{I_g}{\bar{y}A}.$

Example

A gravity dam is shown below:

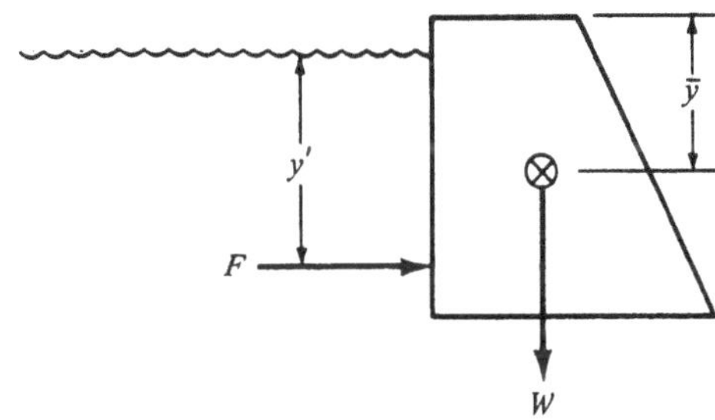

It is important to know F and y' so that the dam can be designed not to tip.

PROBLEMS

1. In the 6-ft-wide watergate shown below, what is the force on the gear teeth of the opening mechanism?

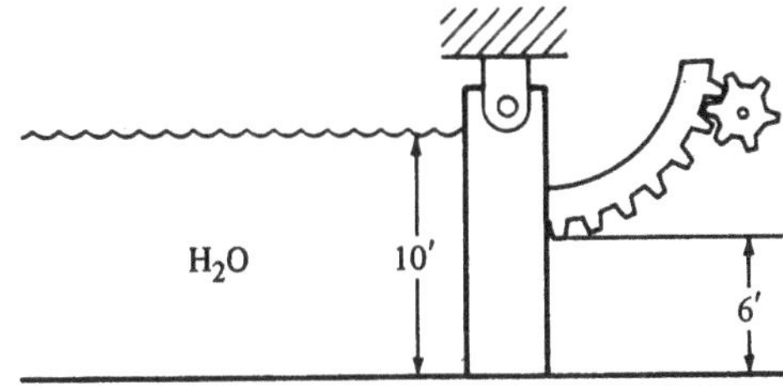

a. 18,720 lb. c. 20,811 lb. e. 36,144 lb.
b. 31,216 lb. d. 16,416 lb.

2. Atmospheric pressure of 29.6 in. Hg will deflect a water manometer how far?

   a. 14.7 ft. c. 32.0 ft. e. 33.5 ft.
   b. 28.9 ft. d. 26.7 ft.

Check your answers.

Answers

1. b.
2. e.
   The density of mercury is 847 lb/ft^3.

C. BUOYANCY

Buoyant forces result from unopposed hydrostatic forces. For example, in a boat water is displaced by air. The hydrostatic forces upward on the boat are opposed by the hydrostatic forces downward due to the air in the boat, which has negligible density compared to water.

Buoyant Force

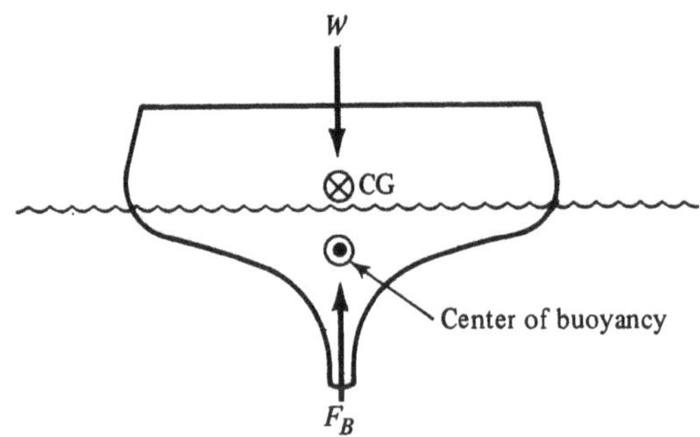

In equilibrium,

$$W = wV$$
$$= F_B,$$

where V is the volume of fluid displaced, W is the weight of the object, and F_B is the buoyant force. The center of buoyancy is the center of gravity of the displaced fluid. Note how moments would develop if the center of buoyancy is not below the center of gravity.

The above relationship is called Archimedes' Principle. It works exactly the same for balloons except that the weight of the gas (helium) displacing the air is not negligible.

> Archimedes' Principle:
>
> $$W = wV,$$
>
> where
>
> wV = Buoyant Force
> w = density of displaced fluid
> V = volume of fluid displaced.

Example

What is the submerged volume of an iceberg with specific gravity 0.9 when floating in seawater with specific gravity of 1.03?

Weight of iceberg = $V_i(62.4)(0.9)$.

Weight of water displaced = $V_w(62.4)(1.03)$.

The weight of the entire iceberg equals the weight of the displaced water, so that

$$V_i(62.4)(0.9) = V_w(62.4)(1.03)$$

and

$$\frac{V_w}{V_i} = \frac{(62.4)(0.9)}{(62.4)(1.03)} = 0.874.$$

The iceberg is 87.4% submerged.

PROBLEMS

1. What is the buoyant force on a $\frac{1}{8}''$ bubble in water?

   a. 3.0×10^{-4} lb. c. 11.8×10^{-4} lb. e. 2.6×10^{-4} lb.
   b. 3.7×10^{-5} lb. d. 3.9×10^{-4} lb.

2. A piece of material weighing 9 lb weighs 5.32 lb when submerged in water. Its density is:

   a. 70 lb/ft^3. c. 162 lb/ft^3. e. 279 lb/ft^3.
   b. 96 lb/ft^3. d. 153 lb/ft^3.

Check your answers.

Answers

1. b.
2. d.

D. FLUID KINEMATICS

Kinematics include those cases where the kinetic energy term in the Bernoulli Equation is not zero. This implies flow:

$$Q = wAv(\text{lb/sec}).$$

The continuity equation is a conservation of mass equation. It simply says that in a conduit flow is constant.

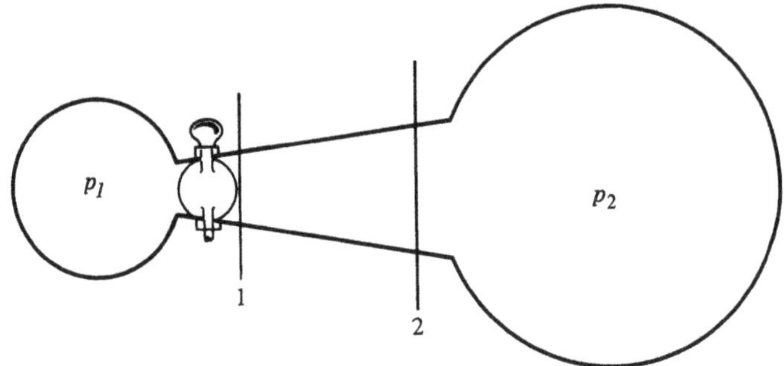

Consider that $p_1 > p_2$ when the valve is opened. The continuity equation is

$$Q = w_1 A_1 v_1 = w_2 A_2 v_2,$$

where

w = density in lb/ft^3;
A = area in ft^2;
v = velocity in ft/sec;
$w_1 = w_2$ for incompressible fluids.

Kinetic energy is measured by the *pitot tube*, a device which converts kinetic energy into gradient energy.

Velocity–Pitot Tube

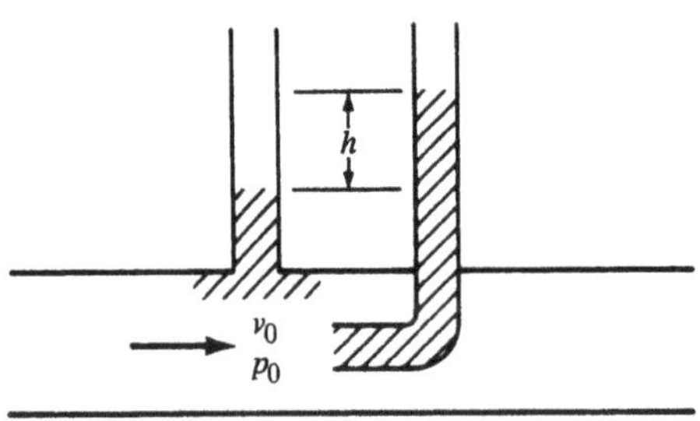

Applying the Bernoulli Equation,

$$v_0 = \sqrt{2gh}.$$

The two main flow regulating devices in hydraulic systems are the *nozzle* or *orifice* in *closed systems* and the *weir* in *open systems.*

Flow Measurement–Orifices

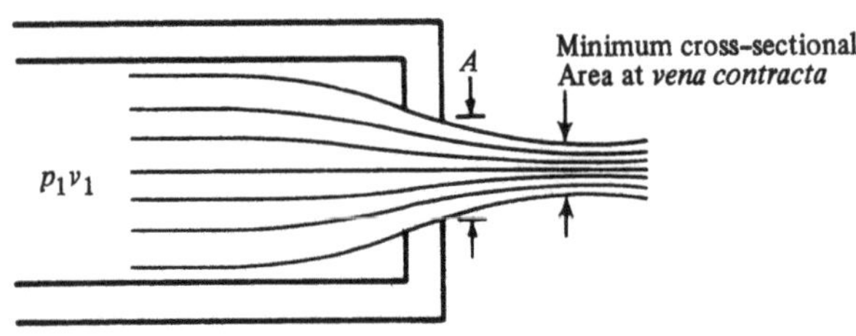

$$v = C_v \sqrt{2g\left[\frac{p_1}{w} + \frac{v_1^2}{2g}\right]}$$

C_v = velocity coefficient
(dependent on friction)

$Q = wC_c Av$

C_c = coefficient of contraction
(dependent on the vena contracta)

$$Q = C_d wA \sqrt{2g\left[\frac{p_1}{w} + \frac{v_1^2}{2g}\right]}$$

C_d = coefficient of discharge

$C_d = C_v C_c$.

The only difference between an orifice and a nozzle is that the stream is unconstrained by an orifice while a nozzle is shaped to accommodate the streamlines. The *vena contracta* of a nozzle is its minimum cross-sectional area.

Weirs

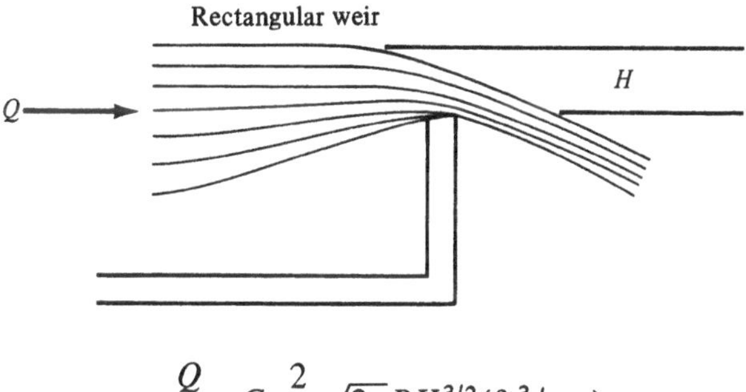

$$\frac{Q}{w} = C_d \frac{2}{3} \sqrt{2g} BH^{3/2} (\text{ft}^3/\text{sec})$$

B = width of weir.

Both the orifice and the weir are devices for converting potential energy into kinetic energy.

Kinetic-Energy Conversions:
Pitot Tube:
$V = \sqrt{2gh}$;
Orifice:
$V = \sqrt{2g\left[\frac{p_1}{w} + \frac{v_1^2}{2g}\right]}$;
Rectangular Weir:
$Q/w = \frac{2}{3}\sqrt{2g} BH^{3/2}$.

Example

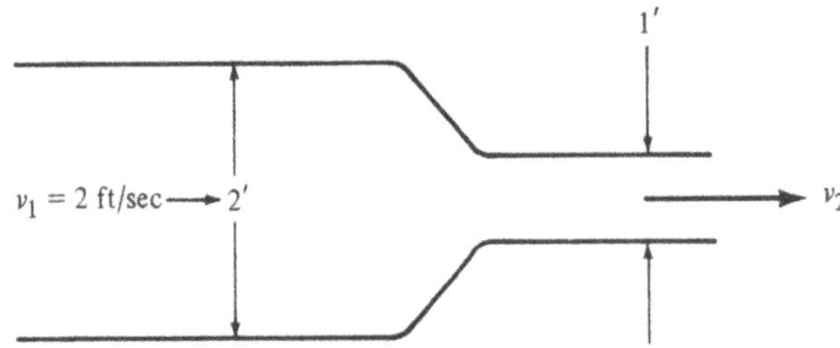

The continuity equation allows us to calculate the final velocity for this incompressible fluid:

$$v_1 A_1 = v_2 A_2$$

$$v_2 = v_1 \frac{A_1}{A_2} = 2\frac{\pi(1)^2}{\pi(\frac{1}{2})^2} = 8 \text{ ft/sec.}$$

The flow rate if the fluid is water is

$$Q = wAv = (62.4)(\pi)(1)^2(2) = 392 \text{ lb/sec.}$$

PROBLEMS

1. In the diagram below, what is the pressure drop from 1 to 2?

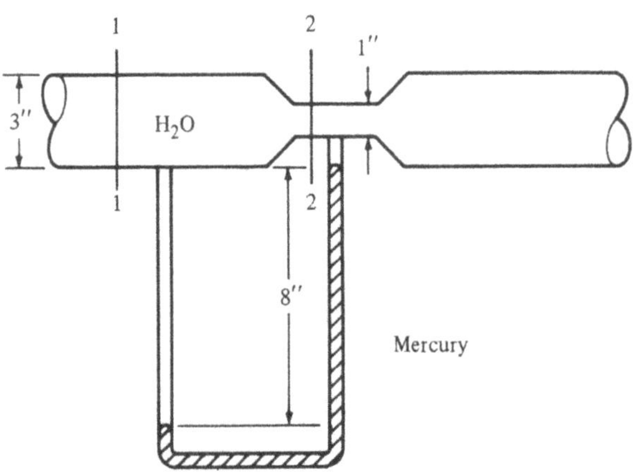

a. 262 psf. c. 350 psf. e. 524 psf.
b. 468 psf. d. 623 psf.

2. In the venturi nozzle above, what is the initial velocity at station 1?

a. 1.64 ft/sec. c. 2.60 ft/sec. e. 1.25 ft/sec.
b. 0.29 ft/sec. d. 8.33 ft/sec.

Check your answers.

Answers

1. e.
2. c.

E. FLUID VISCOSITY

The flow characteristics of a viscous fluid are described by the *Reynolds Number*, a dimensionless number which determines the conditions of flow for any viscous fluid. One condition of flow is *laminar flow*, which has a velocity gradient across the conduit. The velocity of the fluid at the wall of the conduit is small, while maximum velocity occurs at the center of the conduit.

The other type of flow is *turbulent flow*, in which the velocity of fluid is constant across the conduit. The Reynolds Number is defined for a circular conduit flowing full. For conduits of other shapes or for conduits which are not full, the *Hydraulic Radius* is the equivalent parameter. The Hydraulic Radius is defined as the cross-sectional area of the fluid divided by the wetted perimeter.

Reynolds Number:

$$N_R = \frac{Dv\rho}{\mu},$$

where
D = diameter, ft;
v = velocity, ft/sec;
ρ = density, lb/ft^3;
μ = viscosity, lb/ft-sec.

$N_R < 2000$ laminar flow
$N_R > 2000$ turbulent flow

Hydraulic Radius:

$$R = \frac{A}{P},$$

where
A = cross-sectional area;
P = wetted perimeter.
For Reynolds Number calculations, $4R = D$.

Example

Find the Reynolds Number of oil flowing at 1.77 ft/sec in a 4-inch pipe. The kinematic viscosity is 8.36×10^{-4} ft^2/sec. Is the flow laminar or turbulent?

Definition of kinematic viscosity:

$$\nu = \frac{\mu}{\rho}.$$

Therefore,

$$N_R = \frac{vD}{\nu}$$

$$= \frac{(1.77)(4)}{8.36 \times 10^{-4}} = 707.$$

The flow is laminar.

PROBLEMS

1. Water at 60°F is flowing in the channel shown at 8 ft/sec. What is the nearest Reynolds Number?

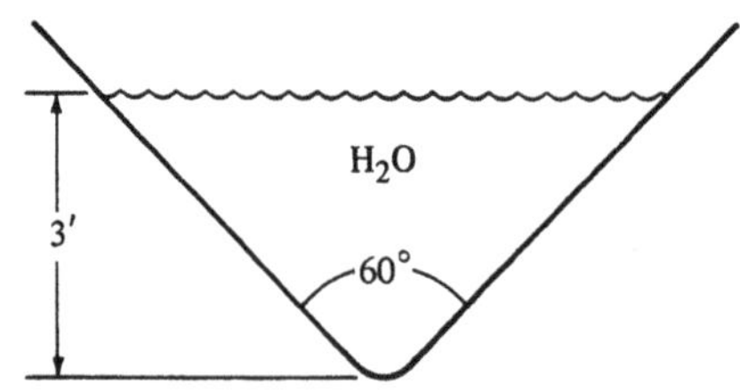

a. 1×10^4. c. 5×10^5. e. 4×10^6.
b. 9×10^5. d. 2×10^6.

2. Which of the following are units of absolute viscosity?

a. Centipoise. c. Stoke. e. Poiseuille.
b. lb/ft^2-second. d. Ft^2/sec.

Check your answers.

Answers

1. d.
   Look up the viscosity of water in a handbook.
2. a.
   Use an index or a set of conversion tables.

F. FRICTION ENERGY

The amount of energy or head lost in a conduit due to friction is determined by relating the Reynolds Number to another dimensionless number called the *friction factor.* These two dimensionless numbers are independent of the fluid or its characteristics, but they are dependent on the internal roughness of the conduit. A plot of these numbers is called the *Moody Diagram* (L. F. Moody, Transactions of the *ASME*, 1944, p. 671.)

You should obtain a Moody Diagram from a textbook or handbook to work fluid problems.

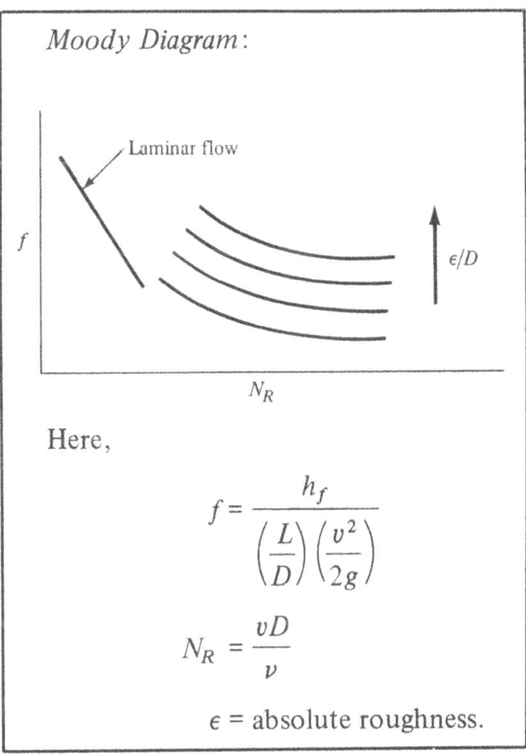

Example A

What is the head loss due to friction of a fluid flowing at 4 ft/sec in a 6-in. pipe 20 ft long with Reynolds number 10^5 (relative roughness = 0.002)?

The friction factor read off the Moody Diagram is $f = 0.025$. Then

$$h_f = f\left(\frac{L}{D}\right)\left(\frac{v^2}{2g}\right)$$

$$= 0.025\left(\frac{20}{\frac{1}{2}}\right)\left(\frac{4^2}{2g}\right)$$

$$= 0.248 \text{ ft.}$$

Example B

What size pipe will be required to transport 2 ft^3/sec of oil with a drop in pressure of 1 psi/1000 ft of pipe? The specific gravity is 0.85, and the absolute viscosity is 12 centipoise at a temperature of 70°F. Assume the pipe is steel.

$$h_f = f\frac{Lv^2}{2gD},$$

where h_f is measured in feet of fluid flowing:

$$h_f = \frac{1 \times 144 \text{ lb/ft}^2}{62.4 \times 0.85 \text{ lb/ft}^3} = 2.72 \text{ ft}/1{,}000 \text{ ft}$$

$$\frac{2gh}{L} = \frac{2g \times 2.72}{1{,}000} = 0.175 = f\frac{v^2}{D}.$$

Now, determine the Reynolds number.

$$\mu = \frac{0.12 \text{ poise}}{478} = 2.50 \times 10^{-4} \text{ lb/ft-sec}$$

$$N_R = \frac{\rho D v}{\mu} = \frac{62.4 \times 0.85}{32.2} \times \frac{1}{2.50 \times 10^{-4}} \times Dv = 6{,}589 Dv.$$

$$2 \text{ ft}^3/\text{sec} = Q = vA = v\pi D^2/4.$$

Giving $vD^2 = 2.55$. These three relationships reduce to

$$N_R = \frac{16{,}800}{D} \quad \text{and} \quad f = 0.0269 D^5.$$

Using the curve for steel pipe from a handbook, $\epsilon/D = 0.00015$ if D is 1 ft,

$$N_R = 16{,}800$$

and

$$f = 0.027.$$

So D should be slightly larger than 1 ft to satisfy the requirements exactly.

PROBLEMS

1. In laminar flow, all of the statements below are correct *except*:

   a. The Reynolds Number increases proportional to velocity.
   b. Friction increases with the roughness of a pipe.
   c. Head loss due to friction is inversely proportional to diameter.
   d. If kinematic viscosity is decreased, the Reynolds Number is increased.
   e. The friction factor is equal to $64/N_R$.

2. What is the Reynolds number for a pipe with characteristics listed below?

$$L/D = 400.$$
$$V = 2 \text{ ft/sec}.$$
$$h_f = 1 \text{ ft}.$$
$$\epsilon/D = 0.008.$$

   a. 1500. c. 2000. e. a or b.
   b. 15000. d. b or c.

Check your answers.

Answers

1. b.
2. e.

G. HYDRODYNAMICS

Hydrodynamics applies where flowing fluid exerts a force on its surroundings. The mechanism for doing this is a transfer of momentum to hydraulic impulse.

> Impulse equals momentum.
>
> $$F\,dt = dmv$$
>
> or
>
> $$F = \frac{dmv}{dt},$$
>
> where
> m = mass in slugs,
> t = seconds,
> v = velocity in ft/sec.
> NOTE: Both $\boldsymbol{F}$ and $\boldsymbol{mv}$ are vector quantities.

Example

What is the force of a stream of water on the flat plate below?

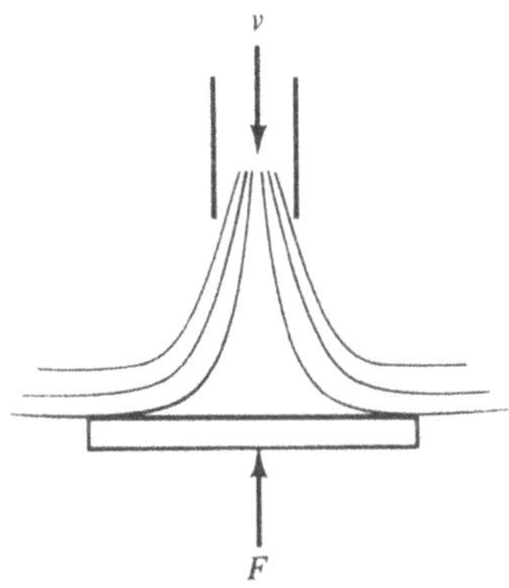

In this case all of the stream's initial momentum is converted to impulse because after impingement there is no component of momentum in the direction of the original momentum.

Therefore,

$$F = \frac{qv}{g},$$

Where
q is in lb/sec,
g is 32.2 ft/sec^2,
v is in ft/sec.

PROBLEMS

1. What is the force in the direction shown on a right elbow with 64.4 lb/sec flowing at 10 ft/sec?

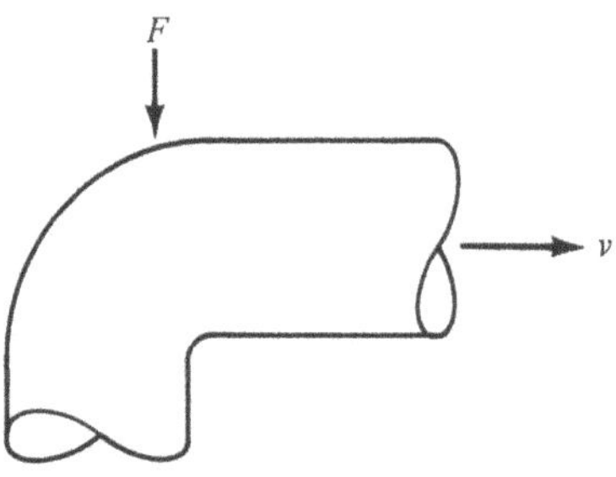

a. 10. c. 30. e. 1288.
b. 20. d. 644.

2. What is the power output of the old-fashioned water wheel below?

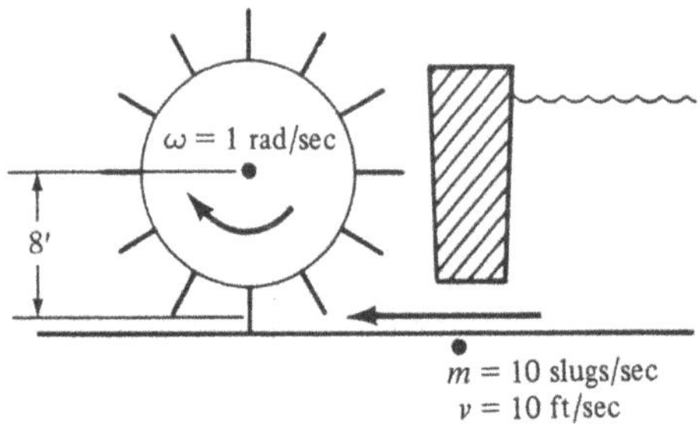

a. 0.66 Hp. c. 1.45 Hp. e. 0.03 Hp.
b. 13.4 Hp. d. 0.29 Hp.

Check your answers.

Answers

1. b.
2. d.
   Use the relative velocity between the stream and the water wheel.

H. AFTERNOON PROBLEM SET

The sketch below shows a wine vat and associated plumbing in a winery.

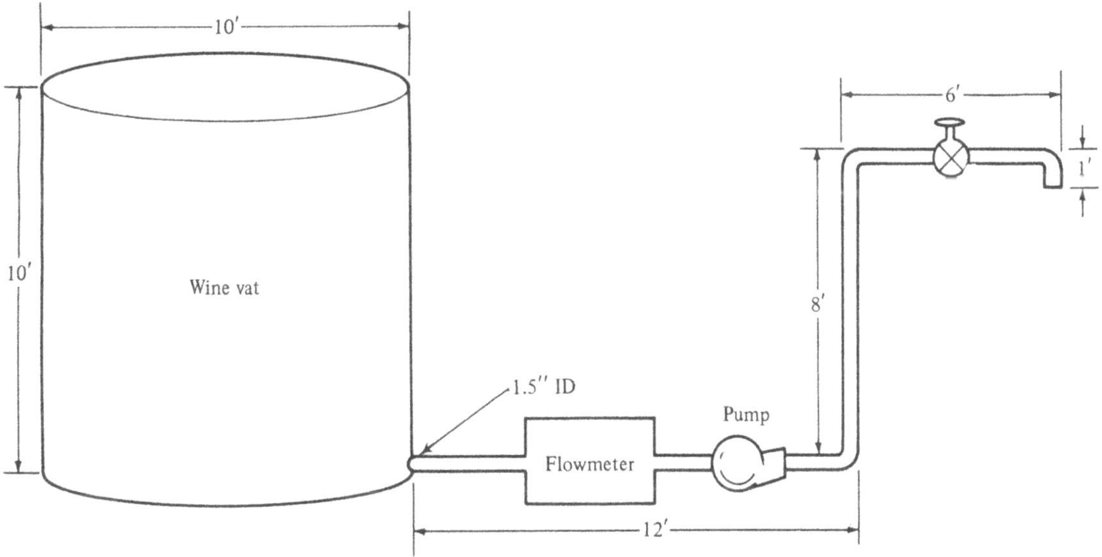

1. With a full tank of wine, a manometer attached to the bottom of the tank shows the following deflection:

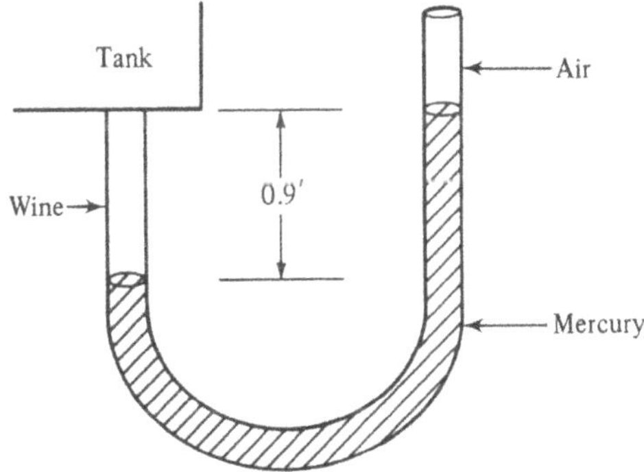

The specific gravity of the wine is:

a. 70. c. 62.4. e. 1.81.
b. 1.12. d. 1.34.

2. The winery chemist determines that the wine is too heavy, so he drains one-fourth of the tank and adds water to replace it. The pressure at the bottom of the tank is now:

a. 68.1 psia. c. 13.7 psig. e. 4.7 psig.
b. 68.1 psig. d. 4.7 psia.

3. The vat is made of wood staves with steel hoops. The bottom hoops are spaced 1 foot apart. The hoops are 2.5 inches wide, $\frac{3}{8}$ inch thick, and have an allowable stress of

16,000 psi. What is the maximum specific gravity the wine can have and still have a factor of safety of 2 for the vat?

a. 2.40. c. 3.75. e. 2.73.
b. 1.24. d. 1.09.

4. A wine is fortified by removing wine and adding 1000 gal of ethanol with a specific gravity of 0.82. If the original specific gravity of the wine was 1.05, how much deeper will a hydrometer that weighs 0.005 lbs float?

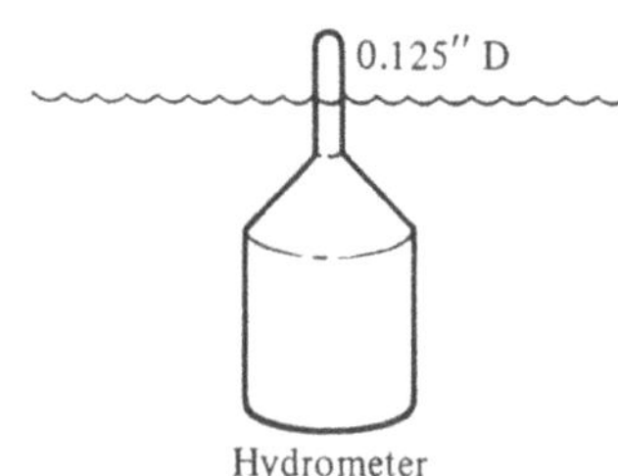

Hydrometer

a. 0.763 in. c. 0.035 in. e. 0.312 in.
b. 0.850 in. d. 0.423 in.

5. When the wine is complete its specific gravity is 1.01. The pump is started. When the tank is nearly empty a flow of 6 gpm is observed. What is the Reynold's Number if the viscosity of the wine is 1.2 centipoises?

a. 63.2×10^4. c. 10.6×10^3. e. 142×10^5.
b. 74.8×10^3. d. 6.2×10^2.

6. The friction factor for pipe with an absolute roughness of 0.0005 is:

a. 0.012. c. 0.034. e. 0.056.
b. 0.022. d. 0.041.

7. What is the horsepower delivered by the pump to the fluid?

a. 0.15. c. 0.001. e. 0.005.
b. 0.20. d. 0.03.

8. If the flow is increased to 6 ft/sec, and the wine still has a specific gravity of 1.01, what axial force will be exerted on the elbow just downstream of the pump? (Assume that the pressure of the fluid at the elbow is 8 psi.)

a. 14.1 lb. c. 8.4 lb. e. 64.2 lb.
b. 168 lb. d. 138 lb.

9. The flowmeter is a venturi meter with a $\frac{3}{4}''$ throat. What is the nearest deflection of a mercury manometer assuming the flow conditions above?

a. 13.6 in. c. 80 in. e. 8.4 in.
b. 103 in. d. 72 in.

10. At the flow conditions above, the valve is closed instantaneously. What is the increased pressure in the line due to water hammer?

    a. 373 psf. c. 53 psf. e. 1081 psf.
    b. 186 psf. d. 786 psf.

Check your answers.

Answers

1. b.
2. e.
3. a.
4. d.
5. c.
6. c.
7. e.
8. d.
9. e.
10. c.

13 Heat Transfer

Chapter Thirteen–Heat Transfer–ID

Discussion of and problems related to conduction, convection, and radiation.

A. CONDUCTION

The rate of heat energy flow depends on a temperature differential and the resistance of the material transmitting the flow. This is analogous to the flow of electricity governed by Ohm's Law:

$$I = E/R$$

where
I is current flow,
E is voltage that causes flow, and
R is resistance.

In heat transfer by conduction, the analogous equation is

$$Q = \frac{KA}{X}\,\Delta T$$

where
Q = rate of heat flow, Btu/hr;
A = area, ft^2;
ΔT = temperature drop, °F;
X = thickness, ft;
K = coefficient of thermal conductivity, Btu/hr ft °F.

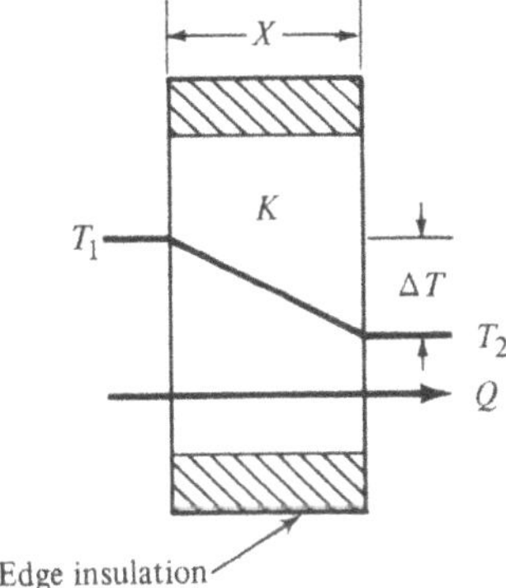

This is called the *Fourier Equation*; it governs heat flow through a homogeneous slab of constant thickness and constant cross-sectional area. By analogy, the term X/KA is called *thermal resistance*:

$$R = \frac{X}{KA}$$

Conduction in a Composite Slab

In a composite slab made up of several different materials, the electrical analogy is that of resistances in series:

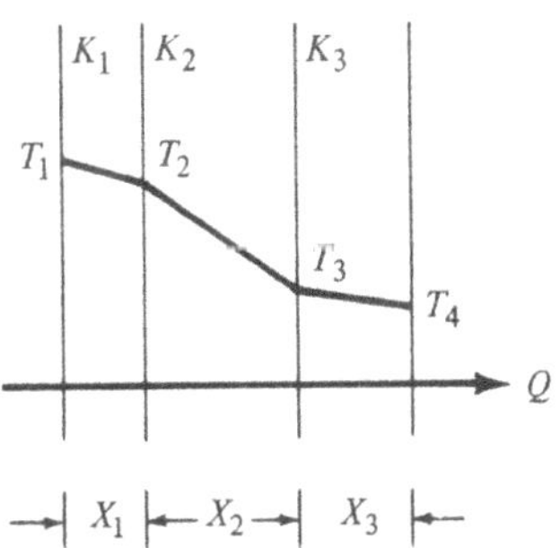

$$Q = \frac{(T_1 - T_4)A}{(\Delta X_1/K_1) + (\Delta X_2/K_2) + (\Delta X_3/K_3)}.$$

Note in the above case that area A is common to all materials; hence the thermal resistances can be written

$$R = \frac{X}{K}.$$

Sometimes the coefficient of thermal conductivity is combined with the thickness to form a term called the *heat transfer coefficient*, U:

$$U = \frac{K}{X} (\text{Btu/hr ft}^2 \text{ °F})$$

Thus the basic conduction equation can be stated in three ways:

$$Q = \frac{KA\,\Delta T}{X}$$

$$Q = UA\,\Delta T$$

$$Q = \frac{A\,\Delta T}{R}.$$

Example

Derive the equation for heat conduction through the wall of a cylindrical pipe:

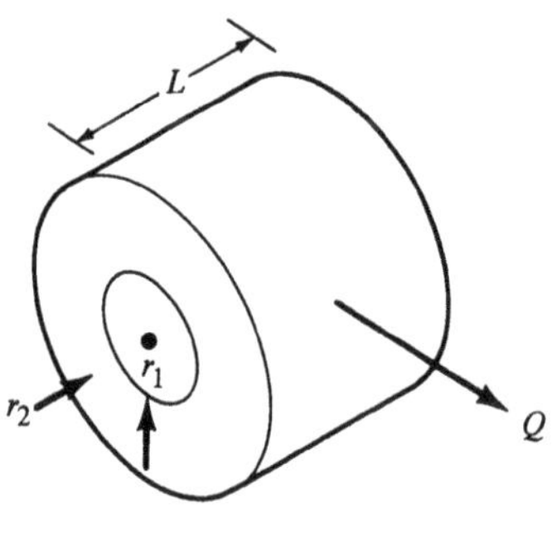

$$Q = KA\frac{\Delta T}{\Delta X}.$$

Note that the cross-sectional area is not constant, but is a function of r. Therefore

$$Q = KL2\pi r\,\frac{dT}{dr}$$

$$\frac{Q\,dr}{r} = KL2\pi\,dT.$$

Integrate both sides:

$$Q\int_{r_1}^{r_2}\frac{dr}{r} = KL2\pi\int_{T_1}^{T_2} dt$$

$$Q = \frac{KL2\pi(T_1 - T_2)}{\ell n\,(r_2/r_1)}.$$

PROBLEMS

1. Given a temperature difference across a wall, the heat flow is:

   a. Directly proportional to the area of the wall and inversely proportional to the thermal resistance.

b. Directly proportional to the heat transfer coefficient and inversely proportional to the temperature difference.
c. Directly proportional to the temperature difference and thickness and inversely proportional to the coefficient of heat transfer.
d. Directly proportional to the thermal resistance and temperature difference.
e. Independent of area.

2. A wall is made of concrete blocks and insulation:

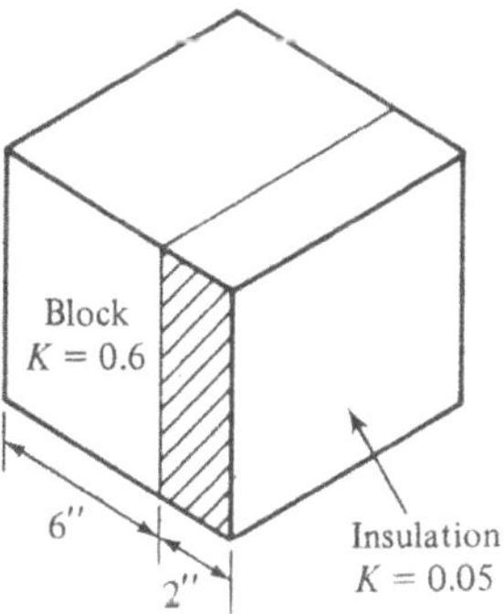

The overall heat transfer coefficient U is:

a. 0.75.
b. 1.50.
c. 1.25.
d. 0.24.
e. 8.00.

Check your answers.

Answers

1. a.
2. d.

B. CONVECTION

A film of fluid such as air adjacent to a heat transfer fluid also inhibits heat flow. The thickness of such a stream of air will depend on wind velocity and other factors and, in any case, is indeterminate.

This is handled by combining the coefficient of heat transfer with the thickness and using the temperature of air far enough out to include all of the temperature gradient. The Fourier Equation for convective heat transfer is:

$$Q = hA(T_s - T_\infty),$$

where
h = convective heat transfer coefficient, Btu/hr ft^2 °F;
T_s = surface temperature;
T_∞ = temperature of air not affected by the surface.

Example

What is the rate of heat flow per unit area through the wall shown below?

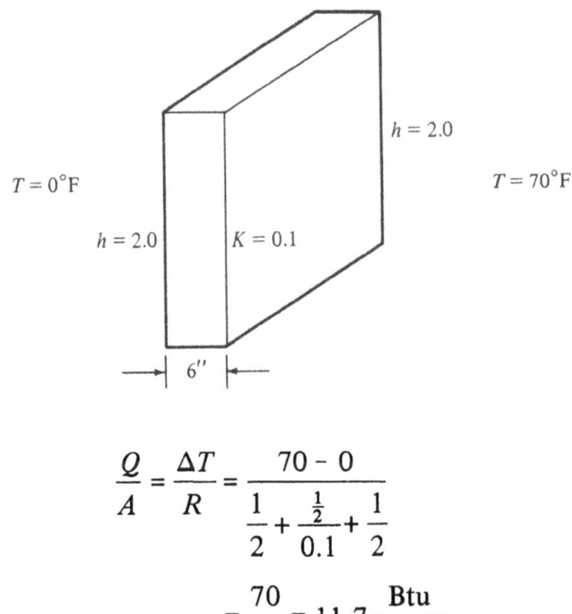

$$\frac{Q}{A} = \frac{\Delta T}{R} = \frac{70 - 0}{\frac{1}{2} + \frac{\frac{1}{2}}{0.1} + \frac{1}{2}}$$

$$= \frac{70}{6} = 11.7 \frac{\text{Btu}}{\text{hr ft}^2}.$$

PROBLEMS

1. Which of the following is *not* a legitimate heat transfer coefficient?

a. $\frac{\text{Btu}}{\text{hr ft °F}}$.

b. $\frac{\text{Btu}}{\text{hr ft}^2\text{ °R}}$.

c. $\frac{\text{W}}{\text{m}^2\text{ °C}}$.

d. $\frac{\text{W}}{\text{hr m}^2\text{ °K}}$.

e. $\frac{\text{J}}{\text{hr m}^2\text{ °C}}$.

2. Fifteen Btu/hr ft² is flowing through the wall of the tank shown below. What must the water temperature be?

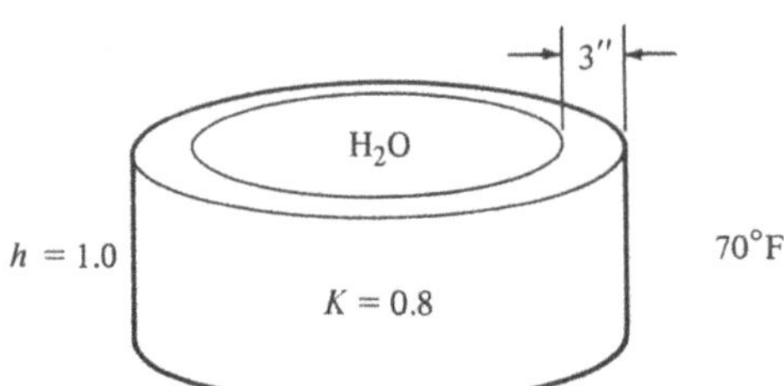

a. 148.
b. 118.
c. 205.
d. 63.
e. 98.

Check your answers.

Answers

1. d.
2. b.

C. RADIATION

Energy can be transmitted from one body to another by electromagnetic radiation. Visible light is an example of such an energy flow.

The ability of a body to emit or receive radiation depends on a property called *emissivity.* Emissivity depends on the frequency of the electromagnetic waves. A perfect black body has an emissivity of unity. It looks black because it is absorbing all visible light and reflecting none. Conversely, a perfect mirror has an emissivity of zero. Stefan and Boltzmann developed the relationship governing heat flow by radiation:

Stefan–Boltzmann Law:

$$Q = A\sigma \frac{(T_1^4 - T_2^4)}{(1/\epsilon_1) + (1/\epsilon_2) - 1},$$

where
T = absolute temperature, °R;
A = area;
$\sigma = 0.1714 \times 10^{-8}$ Btu/ft² hr °R⁴;
ϵ = emissivity ($0 \leqslant \epsilon \leqslant 1$).

Example

What is the flux density of energy traveling between two black balls, one at 70°F and one at 120°F?

$$\frac{Q}{A} = \frac{(0.1714 \times 10^{-8})(580^4 - 530^4)}{\frac{1}{1} + \frac{1}{1} - 1}$$

$$= 59.99 \text{ Btu/hr ft}^2.$$

PROBLEM

A furnace has a wall area of 60 ft². A perfectly emitting flame at 2500°F transfers 100,000 Btu/hr to the furnace wall by radiation. What is the furnace wall temperature?

a. 2480°F.
b. 2490°F.
c. 2860°F.
d. 2020°F.
e. 2750°F.

Check your answer.

Answer

b.

D. AFTERNOON PROBLEM SET

An indoor kiln is constructed of 12″ cement blocks ($K = 0.3$ Btu/hr ft °F) lined with 3″ firebricks ($K = 2.5$ Btu/hr ft °F). Under operation the inner wall temperature is 600°F. The convective heat transfer coefficient at the outer wall is 4.0 Btu/hr ft² °F.

1. The overall heat transfer coefficient of the above kiln is:

   a. 0.660 Btu/hr ft² °F.
   b. 0.333 Btu/hr ft² °F.
   c. 3.68 Btu/hr ft² °F.
   d. 2.28 Btu/hr ft² °F.
   e. 0.272 Btu/hr ft² °F.

2. Heat loss per unit area due to conduction and convection is:

   a. 288 Btu/hr ft².
   b. 144 Btu/hr ft².
   c. 216 Btu/hr ft².
   d. 432 Btu/hr ft².
   e. 72 Btu/hr ft².

3. The inside convective heat transfer coefficient is 2.5 Btu/hr ft² °F. What is the kiln air temperature?

   a. 542°F.
   b. 792°F.
   c. 658°F.
   d. 831°F.
   e. 600°F.

4. Which of the following dimensionless numbers would be used to determine the natural convective heat transfer coefficient?

   a. Prandtl Number.
   b. Reynolds Number.
   c. Gibbs Function.
   d. Lambert's Number.
   e. Hottel Number.

5. The maximum temperature of the cement block is:

   a. 581°F.
   b. 619°F.
   c. 542°F.
   d. 552°F.
   e. 375°F.

6. The outside surface temperature of the kiln is:

   a. 70°F.
   b. 88°F.
   c. 101°F.
   d. 124°F.
   e. 92°F.

7. If the kiln consumes 6.8 kW of power, its log mean surface area is closest to (assume all six sides are of the same construction):

   a. 75 ft^2.
   b. 225 ft^2.
   c. 199 ft^2.
   d. 149 ft^2.
   e. 81 ft^2.

8. What is the equivalent energy input in J/hr?

   a. 3.67×10^5.
   b. 245×10^5.
   c. 9.81×10^4.
   d. 3.413×10^4.
   e. 2.656×10^6.

9. What is the radiation loss per unit area from the outside surface of the kiln to the surrounding room if the surfaces are black?

   a. 75.1 Btu/hr ft^2.
   b. 34.5 Btu/hr ft^2.
   c. 13.9 Btu/hr ft^2.

d. 158.3 Btu/hr ft^2.
e. 14.3 Btu/hr ft^2.

10. What is the approximate percentage change in the number above (#9) if it was determined that both surfaces reflect 10% of incident light?

    a. 10% increase.
    b. 10% decrease.
    c. 20% increase.
    d. 20% decrease.
    e. No change.

Check your answers.

Answers

1. e.
2. b.
3. c.
4. a.
5. a.
6. c.
7. d.
8. b.
9. b.
10. d.

14 Statics

Discussion of and problems related to vector addition; moments and couples; centroids, centers of gravity, and moments of inertia; and trusses.

A. INTRODUCTION

Newton's Force Law states that forces are related to a rate of change in momentum:

$$F = \frac{d(mv)}{dt},$$

where

m = mass in slugs,

v = velocity in ft/sec.

A system in static equilibrium, by definition, has no rate of change of momentum. In other words, a constant-mass system in static equilibrium has either a constant velocity or no velocity. This also implies that the net force on the system is zero.

Since force is a vector quantity, the net force consists of the vector sum of all forces on the system.

An unbalanced linear force will cause linear velocity changes, one mode of motion. The other mode of motion is rotational. The rotational analog of force is the force moment.

Consider the wheel and axle below.

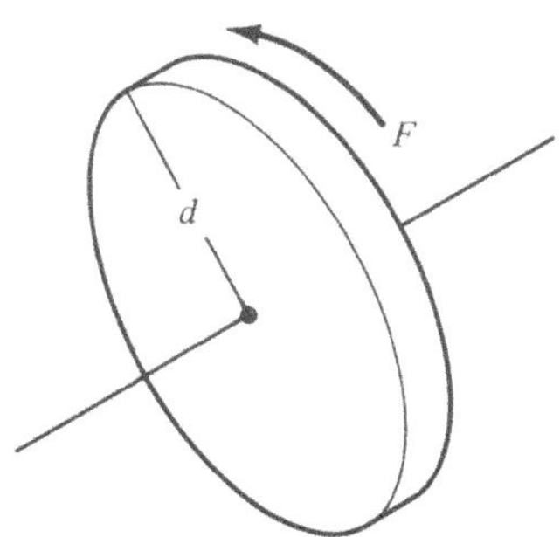

The moment on the wheel about the axle causing a change in rotational velocity is

$$M = Fd.$$

The condition of static equilibrium requires that both the net force and the net moment on a system be zero.

Static Equilibrium:

$$\Sigma F = 0$$

and

$$\Sigma M = 0.$$

NOTE: The sum of the moments about *any* point on or off a body must equal zero.

Example

Consider the simply supported, weightless beam illustrated below:

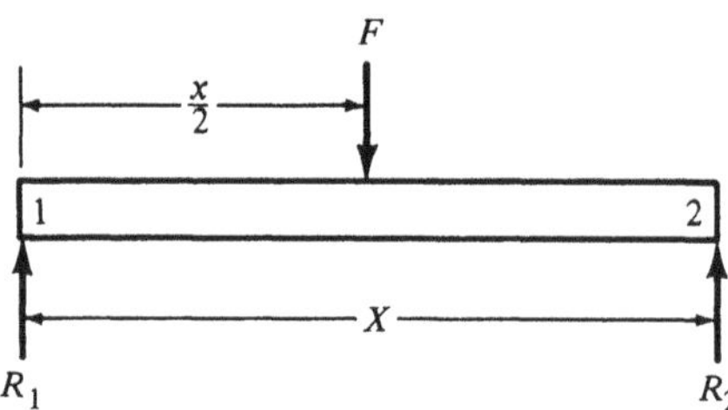

The first condition of static equilibrium yields the equation

$$F = R_1 + R_2.$$

The second condition of static equilibrium yields the following equation when applied to point 1 on the beam:

$$(x)(R_2) = \left(\frac{x}{2}\right)(F)$$

Note that force R_1 plays no part in this equation because the distance between its line of action and point 1 is zero. Hence, the moment due to R_1 is also zero.

Applying the second condition to point 2 yields

$$(x)(R_1) = \left(\frac{x}{2}\right)(F).$$

These applications of the conditions of equilibrium yield three equations in three unknowns. The three equations can be solved simultaneously.

PROBLEMS

1. Which of the systems shown below cannot be in static equilibrium?

a.

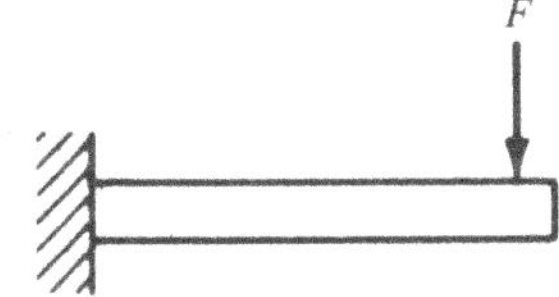

d.

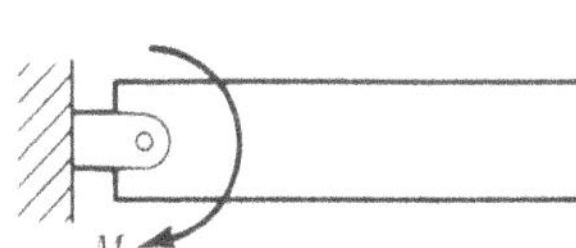

b.

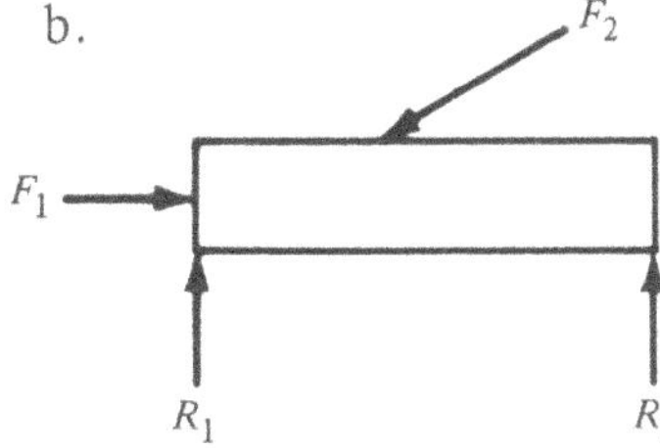

e.

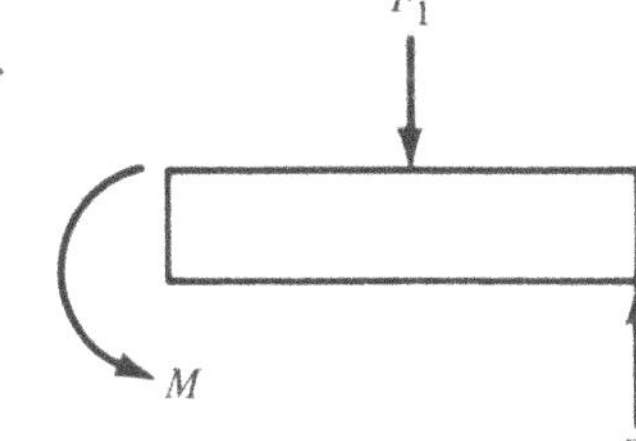

c.

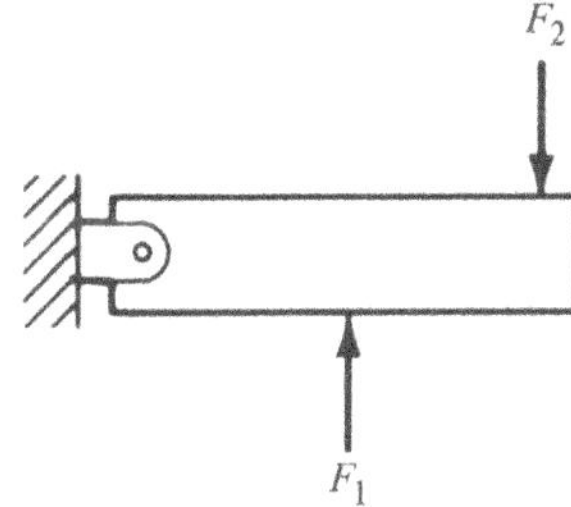

2. What maximum force P can be applied without moving the box shown below?

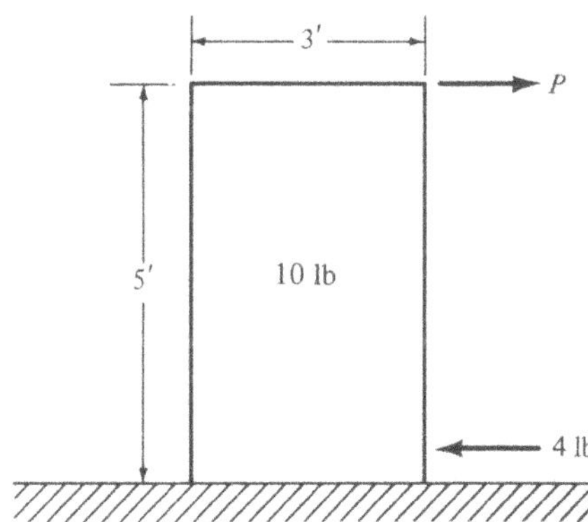

a. 6 lb.
b. 4 lb.
c. 3 lb.
d. 2 lb.
e. 1 lb.

Check your answers.

Answers

1. d.
2. c.

B. VECTOR ADDITION

Since statics is based on net forces and force is a vector quantity, the symbolic methods of adding vectors are important. A vector has both magnitude and direction. The quantity A is identified as a vector by writing it as $\vec{A}$. Graphically, it is shown as

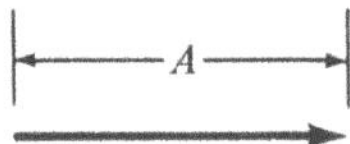

where its magnitude is A, and its direction is that of the arrow.

Vector Addition

Static equilibrium (net force equals zero):

$$\vec{A} + \vec{B} + \vec{E} = 0.$$

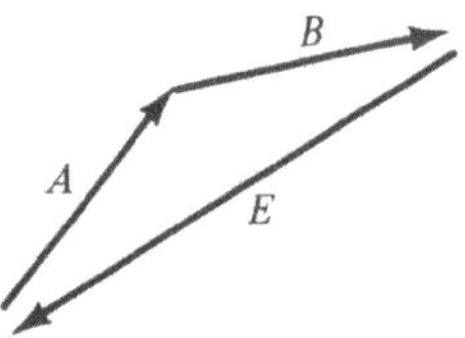

E is called the *equilibrant*. It is the force that opposes A and B. Note the directions of the arrows.

Static inequilibrium (net force not equal to zero):

$$\vec{A} + \vec{B} = \vec{R}.$$

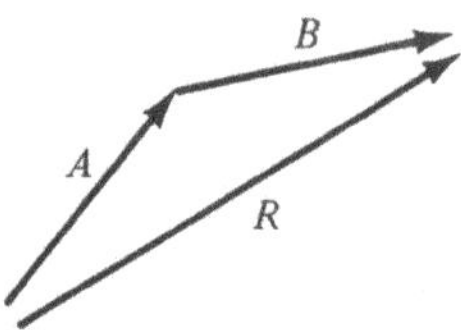

R is called the *resultant* of A and B. It is the vector sum. Again, note the directions of the arrows.

Example

Consider a weightless bar with forces applied as shown below:

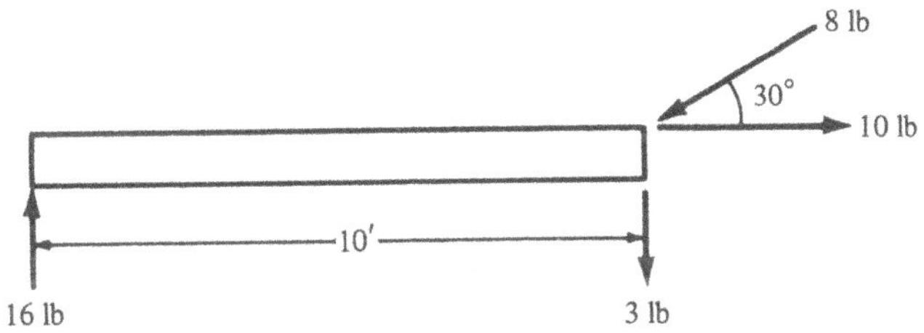

$$\Sigma F_x = 10 - 8 \cos 30 = 10 - 6.92 = 3.08$$

$$\Sigma F_y = 16 - 8 \sin 30 - 3 = 16 - 7 = 9.00.$$

The resultant force on the bar is the vector sum of the above two unbalanced forces:

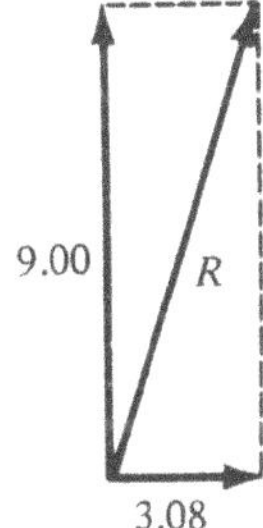

By the Pythagorean Theorem:

$$R = \sqrt{(9.00)^2 + (3.08)^2}$$

$$= \sqrt{90.49}$$

$$= 9.5 \text{ lb.}$$

To achieve static equilibrium, a force of 9.5 lb must be applied to the bar in a direction opposite to the resultant. This is called the *equilibrant*.

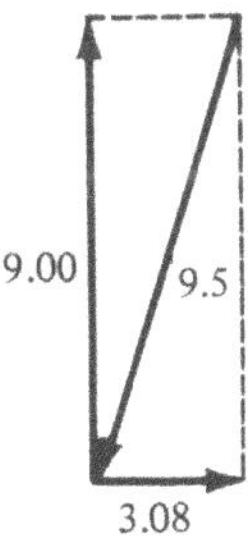

The angle of application is:

$$\theta = \tan^{-1} \frac{9.00}{3.08} = \tan^{-1} 2.92 = 71°.$$

There remains only to find the point of application. This is done through use of the moment equations. First, select an arbitrary point of application a distance x from the left of the bar:

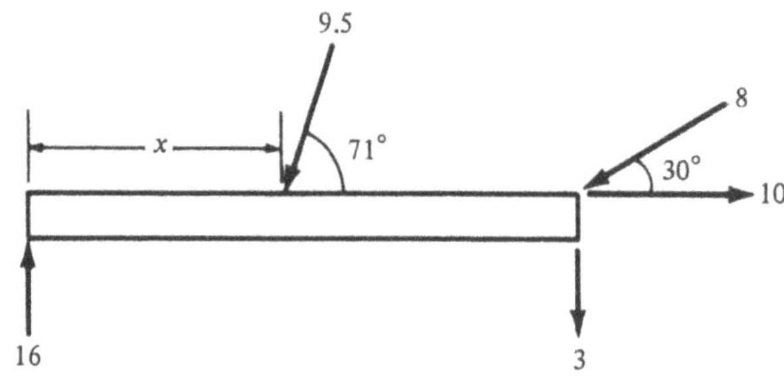

Add the clockwise moments about the left end of the bar and equate to zero:

$$\Sigma M = (9)(x) + (8 \sin 30°)(10) + (3)(10) = 0$$

$$x = -\frac{(7)(10)}{9} = -7.78 \text{ ft.}$$

The negative sign means that the force must be applied 7.78 ft to the left of the left end of the bar.

PROBLEMS

1. The resultant of the force system shown below is:

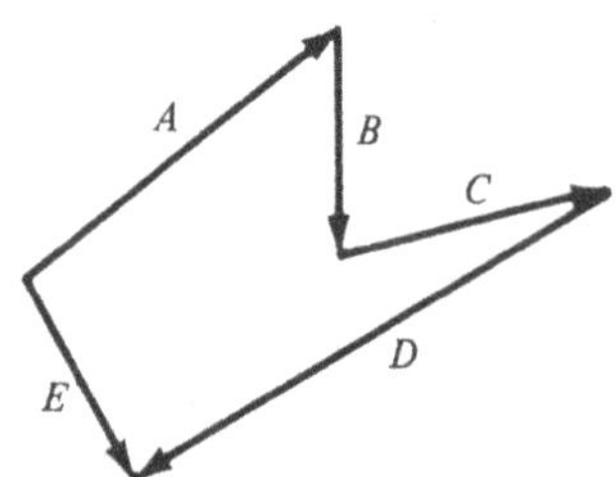

   a. A.
   b. B.
   c. C.
   d. D.
   e. E.

2. The reaction at point 2 due to the 60 lb block shown below is:

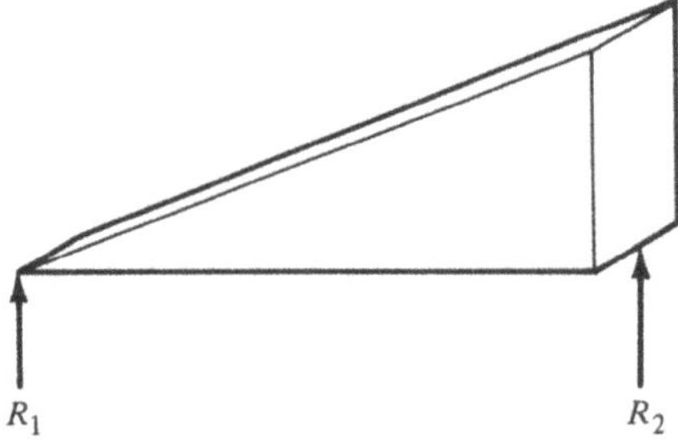

a. 30 lb.
b. 20 lb.
c. 45 lb.
d. 40 lb.
e. 15 lb.

Check your answers.

Answers

1. e.
2. d.

C. MOMENTS AND COUPLES

In static equilibrium the moment about any point must equal zero. A *moment* can be represented by a free-standing moment, as illustrated in a cantilever beam.

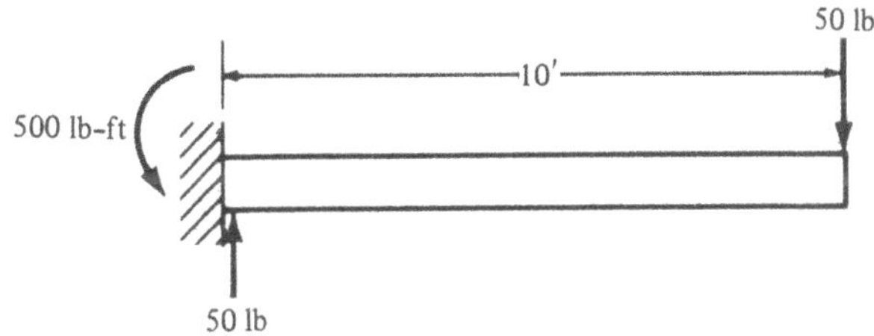

The 500 lb-ft moment which is the net effect of the torsion-resisting capability of the beam support is an entity which can be considered to be any force times distance which equals 500 lb-ft.

A *couple* is the net moment created by two equal but opposite forces with a distance between their lines of action:

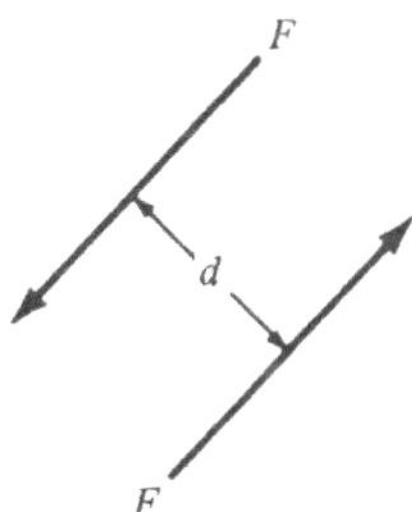

The moment of the above couple is Fd. The effect of a couple is independent of the location on a body.

> A *moment* is the action of a force about a point.
> A *couple* is a moment which is independent of location.

Example

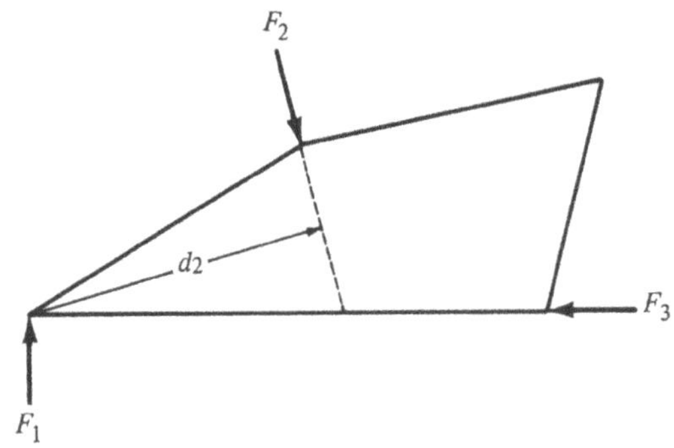

Assume $\vec{F_1} + \vec{F_2} + \vec{F_3} = 0$. Remove F_2 and F_3, and then replace with a moment about point 1. Its magnitude would be $F_2 d_2$. What couple would have the same effect?

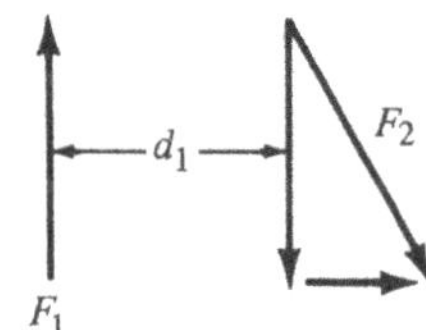

The magnitude of the couple is $F_1 d_1$.

PROBLEM

In the diagram below, if the 40 lb-ft couple is moved to point B, the 10 lb force must be changed to what value to preserve static equilibrium?

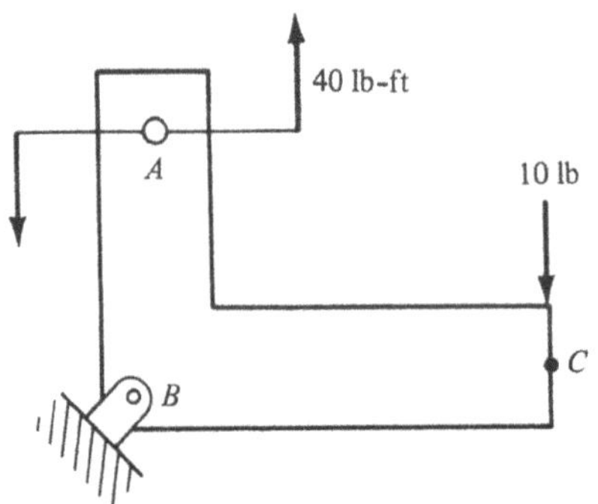

a. 5 lb.
b. 45 lb.
c. 35 lb.
d. 10 lb.
e. 15 lb.

Check your answer.

Answer

d.

D. CENTROIDS, CENTERS OF GRAVITY, AND MOMENTS OF INERTIA

A *centroid* relates to a plane area. The *center of gravity* relates to a mass. The weight of a body can always be assumed to be a point force acting through the center of gravity.

Centroid and Center of Gravity

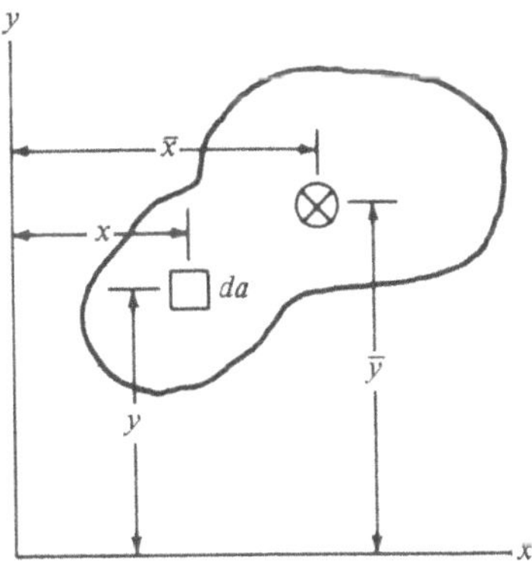

Centroid of Area:

$$\bar{x} = \frac{\int x\, dA}{A}$$

$$\bar{y} = \frac{\int y\, dA}{A}.$$

$\int x\, da$ is called the *moment of the area* with respect to the x-axis.
Center of Gravity of a Mass:

$$\bar{x} = \frac{\int x\, dm}{m}$$

$$\bar{y} = \frac{\int y\, dm}{m}.$$

Centroid of a Composite Area

Consider a square and a semicircle:

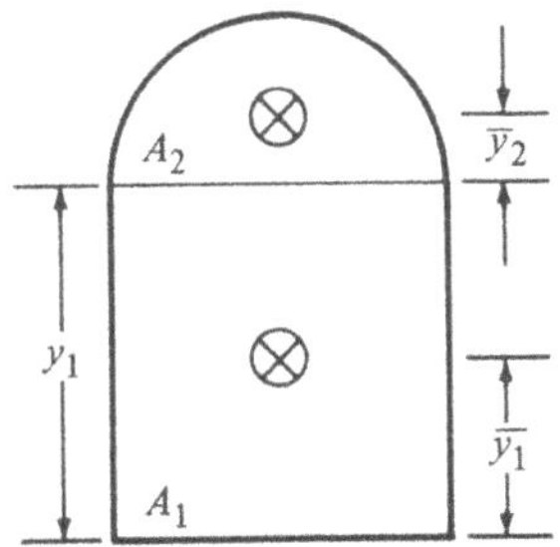

The centroid is

$$\bar{y} = \frac{A_1\bar{y}_1 + A_2(y_1 + \bar{y}_2)}{A_1 + A_2}.$$

If the above represented a cube and a hemisphere, the center of gravity would be:

$$\bar{y} = \frac{m_1\bar{y}_1 + m_2(y_1 + \bar{y}_2)}{m_1 + m_2}.$$

Moments of Inertia

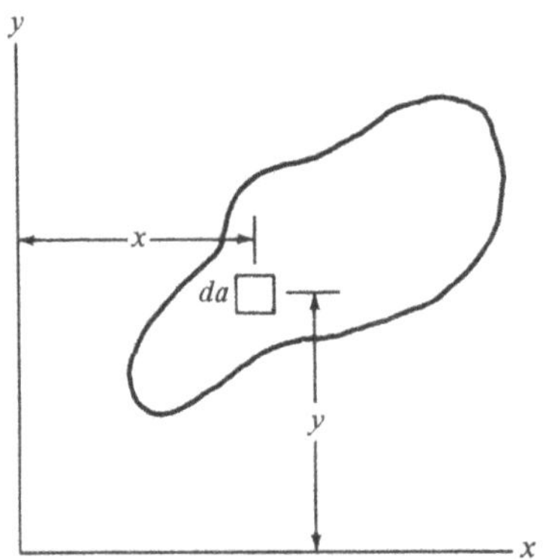

Moment of Inertia (Second Moment) of Area:

$$I_x = \int y^2 \, dA, \qquad I_y = \int x^2 \, dA,$$

units: ft^4

If the figure above represented a mass:

$$I_x = \int y^2 \, dm, \qquad I_y = \int x^2 \, dm,$$

units: slug-ft^2

Parallel-Axis Theorem

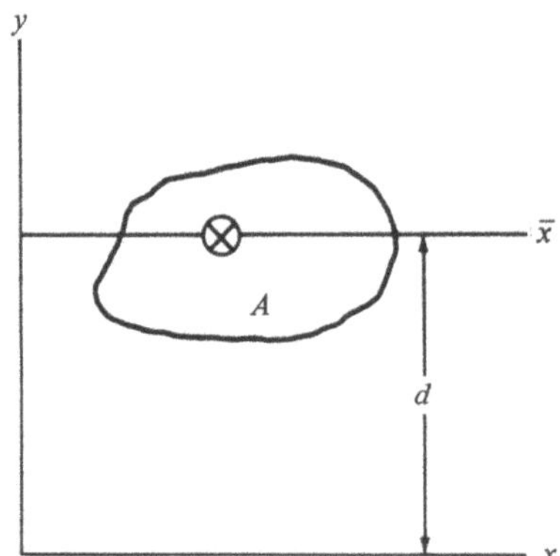

$\bar{x}$ is the axis through the centroid; I_g is the moment of inertia about the centroid.

$$I_x = I_g + Ad^2.$$

Composite Areas–Moment of Inertia

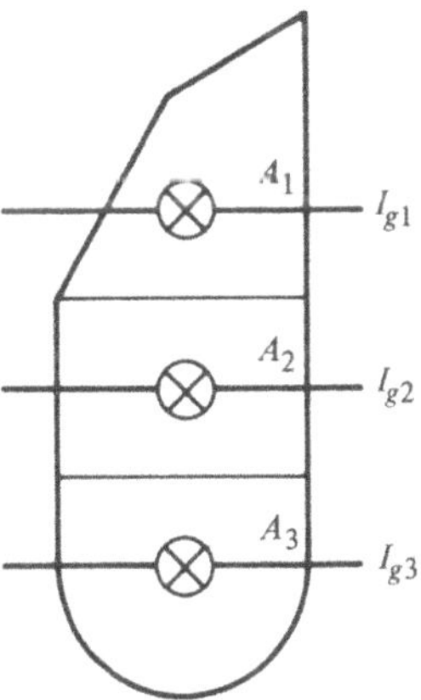

When the moment of inertia of an irregular area made up of several common areas is required, it can be found by considering each common area separately and using the parallel-axis theorem to find the moment of inertia of this area with respect to the given axis. The total I for the entire area will be the sum of the I's of the individual areas with respect to the given axis:

$$I_x = I_{g1} + A_1 d_1^2 + I_{g2} + A_2 d_2^2 + I_{g3} + A_3 d_3^2$$

Centroid:	$\bar{x} = \frac{\int x\, dA}{A}.$
Center of Gravity:	$\bar{x} = \frac{\int x\, dm}{m}.$
Moment of Inertia of an Area:	$I_x = \int y^2\, dA.$
Moment of Inertia of a Mass:	$I_x = \int y^2\, dm.$

Example

Where is the center of gravity and what is the moment of inertia of the two bodies shown on p. 174?

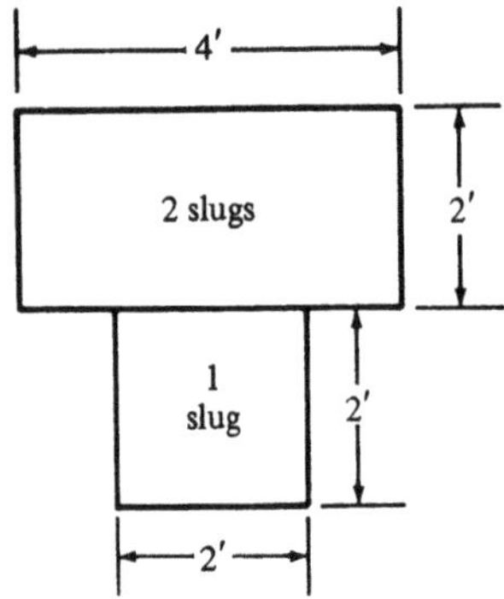

From a handbook:

$$\bar{y} = h/2 = 1$$

$$I_{g1} = \frac{m}{12}(b^2 + h^2) = \frac{1}{12}(2^2 + 2^2)$$

$$\bar{y}_2 = h/2 = 1$$

$$I_{g2} = \frac{m}{12}(b^2 + h^2) = \frac{2}{12}(4^2 + 2^2)$$

The composite center of gravity measured from the base is

$$\bar{y} = \frac{(1)(1) + (1 + 2)(2)}{1 + 2}$$

$$= 2.33 \text{ ft.}$$

The composite moment of inertia about the base is

$$I_x = (1)(1) + \frac{8}{12} + (3)(2) + \frac{40}{12}$$

$$= 11 \text{ slug-ft}^2.$$

PROBLEMS

1. Which of the following units do *not* represent a second moment?

   a. Slug-ft^2.
   b. In^4.
   c. Kg-m-sec^2.
   d. Lb-ft-sec^2.
   e. N-m-sec^2.

2. What is the location of the centroid of the parabola $y^2 = 8x$?

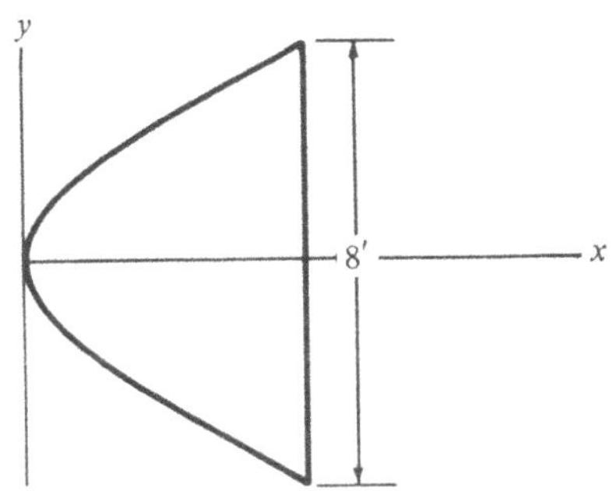

a. 0, 0.8.
b. 0, 1.2.
c. 1.2, 0.
d. 0.8, 0.
e. None of the above.

Check your answers.

Answers

1. c.
2. b.

E. TRUSSES

The truss structure makes use of pin-jointed members like the jib crane shown below:

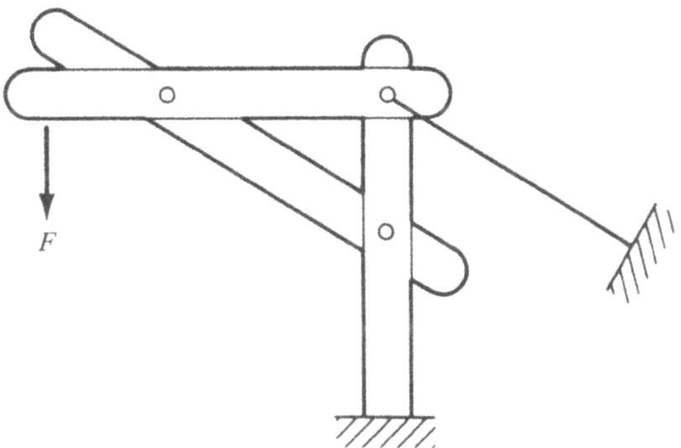

The two methods of analyzing a truss are:

1. Analyze each pin joint by joint, assuming static equilibrium. The nature of a pin joint is such that the joint can exert no moments on the members. Therefore, all members are either in tension or compression only.
2. Consider that since there is no motion of any member with respect to the others, the entire structure can be treated as a free body and the rules of static equilibrium applied.

Bridge Truss

In a truss, the members are force members, either in tension or compression. To find these forces algebraically, two general methods are used. (Reactions are first found, considering the entire truss as a free body.)

Joints—in which the free-body diagram is drawn for each joint and unknowns are found by the equations

$$\Sigma F_x = 0, \quad \Sigma F_y = 0.$$

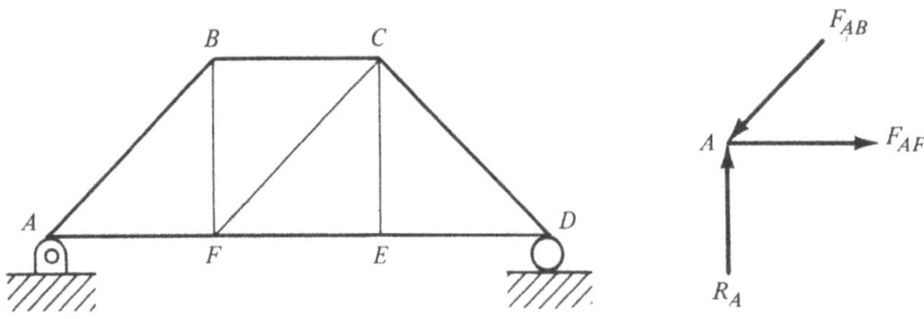

Sections—in which a section is passed, cutting the member for which stress is required. The free body then consists of several joints and members. Required force is one of the external forces on the free body and is found by applying conditions of equilibrium:

$$\Sigma F_x = 0, \quad \Sigma F_y = 0, \quad \Sigma M = 0.$$

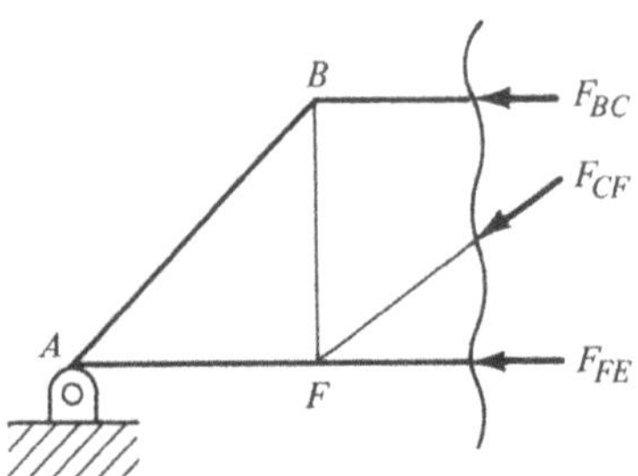

Truss Analysis:

$\Sigma F = 0$ for each joint.

$\Sigma F = 0$ and $\Sigma M = 0$ for the complete truss or portion thereof.

Example

Consider the following bridge truss:

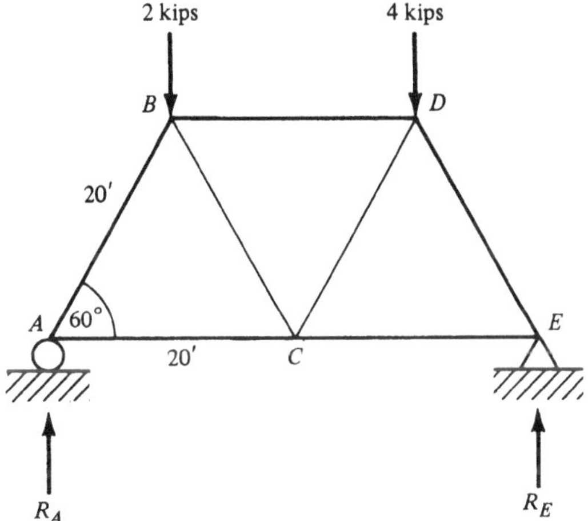

What is the load in member *CD*? First solve for reactions R_A and R_E:

$$\Sigma M_A = 0 = (R_E)(40) - (4000)(30) - (2000)(10),$$

hence $R_E = 3500$ lb.

$$\Sigma M_E = 0 = -(R_A)(40) + (2000)(30) + (4000)(10),$$

hence $R_A = 2500$ lb.

A complete solution would involve looking at each joint:

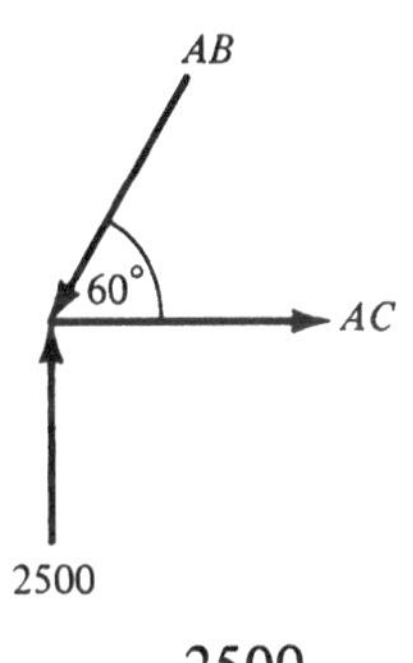

$$AB = \frac{2500}{\sin 60°}$$

$$AC = AB \cos 60°.$$

Going through the truss joint by joint would eventually lead to a solution for *CD*. The free-body method will yield the same result faster.

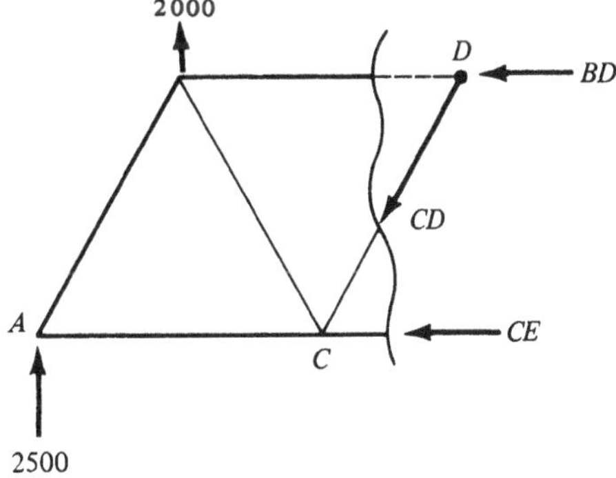

$$\Sigma F_C = 0 = 2500 - 2000 - CD \sin 60$$

$$CD = 577 \text{ lb in the direction shown.}$$

If we desire to find *CE*,

$$\Sigma M_D = 0 = (2500)(30) - (2000)(20) + (CE)(20)(\sin 60).$$

Or, if we desire to find *BD*, we would sum moments about *C*. Note that for any cut through the truss an equation in one unknown can be written to solve for any cut member as long as no more than three members are cut.

PROBLEMS

1. What is the force in section *a* of the weightless truss shown below?

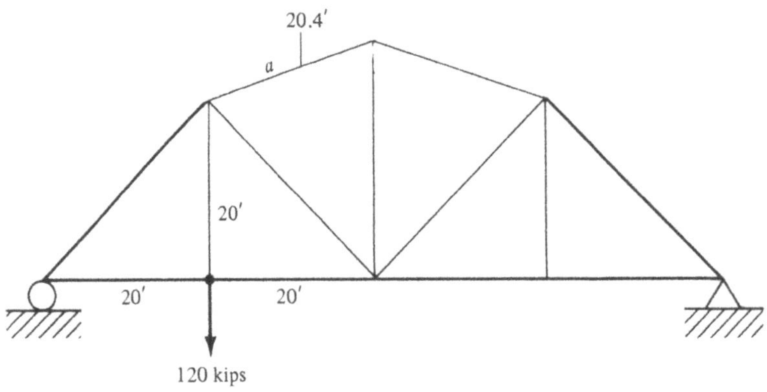

a. 28.3 K tension.
b. 28.3 K compression.
c. 51 K tension
d. 56.6 K tension.
e. 20 K tension.

2. What is the tension in the cable of the truss shown below?

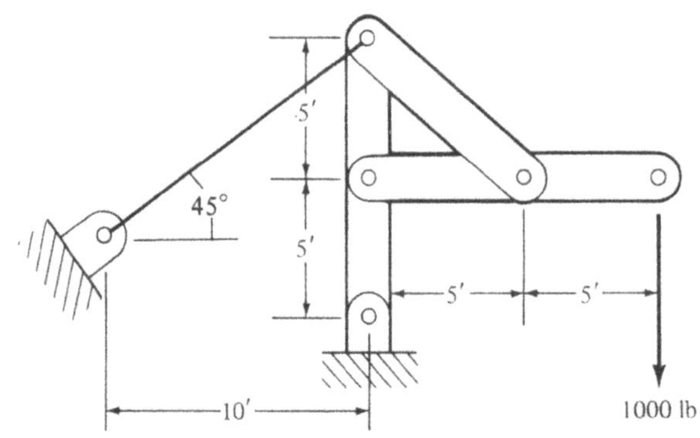

a. 2828 lb.
b. 1413 lb.
c. 2120 lb.
d. 4242 lb.
e. 1060 lb.

Check your answers.

Answers

1. c.
2. b.

F. AFTERNOON PROBLEM SET

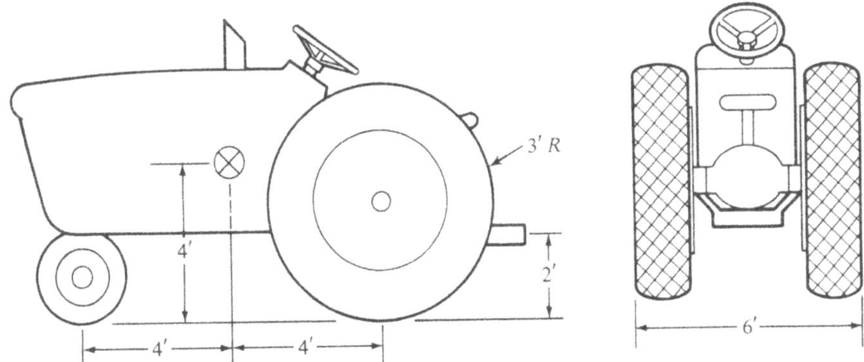

1. What is the maximum safe draw bar pull of the 4000 lb tractor?

   a. 4,000 lb.
   b. 32,000 lb.
   c. 16,000 lb.
   d. 8,000 lb.
   e. None of the above.

2. If the tractor is pulling 1,000 lb, what is the maximum slope that it can safely go up?

   a. 18°.
   b. 40°.
   c. 42°.
   d. 35°.
   e. 38°.

3. If the hitch is raised 1 ft, what is the percentage reduction in tractive force?

   a. 50%.
   b. 66%.
   c. 33%.
   d. 15%.
   e. 10%.

4. What is the slope of the maximum safe side hill the tractor can traverse?

   a. 35°.
   b. 15°.
   c. 48°.
   d. 20°.
   e. 28°.

5. What is the answer to question 4 if 250-lb wheel weights are added to each rear wheel?

   a. 20°.
   b. 22°.
   c. 30°.
   d. 37°.
   e. 40°.

The front-end loader shown below is attached to the tractor:

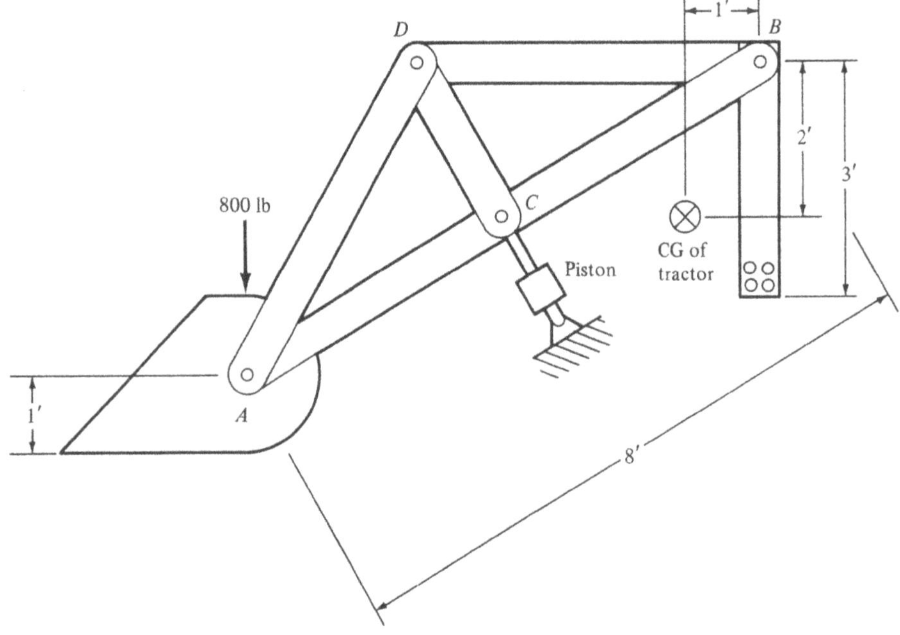

6. What is the pressure in the 4″-diameter piston when the bucket is just leaving the ground?

   a. 25 psi.
   b. 75 psi.
   c. 100 psi.
   d. 125 psi.
   e. 150 psi.

7. What is the nearest force in member *DB* in the piston shown if member *DC* is 24″ long?

   a. 900 lb.
   b. 1000 lb.

c. 1200 lb.
d. 1400 lb.
e. 1600 lb.

8. What is the vertical shearing force in pin *B* in the position shown?

   a. 350 lb.
   b. 400 lb.
   c. 450 lb.
   d. 500 lb.
   e. 550 lb.

9. If the bucket is raised so that *AB* is horizontal, what is the force in member *AD*? (Assume piston force is axial to *DC*.)

   a. 1000 lb.
   b. 1800 lb.
   c. 1600 lb.
   d. 2000 lb.
   e. 1400 lb.

10. In the position shown above, what is the safe drawbar pull if the *CG* of the loader is at pin *C*?

   a. 12,400 lb.
   b. 12,100 lb.
   c. 11,800 lb.
   d. 13,600 lb.
   e. 6,200 lb.

Check your answers.

Answers

1. d.
2. e.
3. c.
4. a.
5. d.
6. c.
7. d.
8. d.
9. b.
10. a.

15 Kinematics and Dynamics

Discussion of and problems related to kinematics, relative kinematics, vector multiplication, forces, centrifugal force, impulse and momentum, and energy.

A. INTRODUCTION

Kinematics and dynamics deal with cases having a change in momentum. Newton's Force Law can be expanded to derive all the relationships of kinematics and dynamics. When dealing with linear momentum, Newton said:

$$F = \frac{d(mv)}{dt}$$

This can be expanded to cover kinematics, dynamics, and momentum.

Kinematics

Kinematics deals with the definition of the motion terms:

$v = dx/dt$ rate of change of distance with respect to time,

$a = dv/dt = \dfrac{d^2x}{dt^2}$ rate of change of velocity with respect to time,

and the analogous rotational terms (θ is in radians):

$\omega = d\theta/dt$ rate of change of angular displacement with respect to time.

$\alpha = d\omega/dt = \dfrac{d^2\theta}{dt^2}$ rate of change of angular velocity with respect to time.

Dynamics

Dynamics deals with forces:

$$F = \frac{d(mv)}{dt} = v\frac{dm}{dt} + m\frac{dv}{dt}.$$

The first term of this relationship is usually zero since mass does not change with respect to time. (Note the exception in a solid-fuel rocket motor.)
In rotational terms, Newton's Law is

$$\tau = \frac{d(I\omega)}{dt},$$

where
τ = torque,
I = moment of inertia,
ω = rotational velocity.

Momentum

Momentum deals with the product mv as a vector entity. The rotational analogue of momentum is $I\omega$.

Newtonian Physics:
$F = \dfrac{d(mv)}{dt}$
$\tau = \dfrac{d(I\omega)}{dt}.$

Example

What torque is required to accelerate a flywheel from 20 rpm to 80 rpm in 30 seconds if the moment of inertia of the flywheel is 800 slug-ft^2?

$$\tau = \frac{d(I\omega)}{dt} = \frac{I}{t}\Delta\omega$$

$$= \frac{800}{30}(80 - 20)\frac{2\pi}{60} = 168 \text{ lb-ft.}$$

PROBLEMS

1. A body is moving such that its position with respect to time is governed by

$$x = 17t^2 - 6t.$$

What is its velocity at $t = 4$ seconds?

a. 59 ft/sec.
b. 71 ft/sec.
c. 130 ft/sec.
d. 136 ft/sec.
e. 142 ft/sec.

2. What is the acceleration of the system shown below?

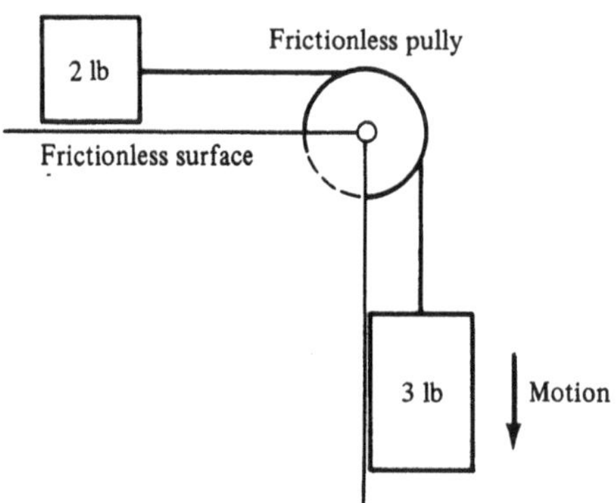

a. 0.2 ft/sec^2.
b. 19.3 ft/sec^2.
c. 1.0 ft/sec^2.
d. 8.6 ft/sec^2.
e. 0.8 ft/sec^2.

Check your answers.

Answers

1. c.
2. b.

B. KINEMATICS

The following kinematic terms can be derived from the basic definitions of displacement, velocity, and acceleration and their rotational analogues.

Kinematics: the study of motion.
Motion of a particle in a straight line:

$$s = \text{linear displacement}$$

$$v = \text{linear velocity} = \frac{ds}{dt}$$

$$a = \text{linear acceleration} = \frac{dv}{dt} = \frac{d^2s}{dt^2} = \ddot{s}.$$

Particle moving in a straight line with constant acceleration:

$$v = v_0 + at$$

$$s = v_0 t + \tfrac{1}{2}at^2$$

$$v^2 = v_0^2 + 2as.$$

Particle moving in a circular path:

$$\theta = \text{angular displacement}$$

$$\omega = \text{angular velocity} = \frac{d\theta}{dt}$$

$$\alpha = \text{angular acceleration} = \frac{d\omega}{dt}.$$

Example

What rotation does a wheel undergo in time t sec after an acceleration α rad/sec^2 and starting with an initial velocity ω rad/sec?

$$\alpha = \frac{d\omega}{dt}, \quad \text{or} \quad d\omega = \alpha\, dt.$$

Therefore,

$$\Delta\omega = \int_1^2 \alpha\, dt$$

$$= \alpha\, \Delta t$$

$$\Delta\omega = \omega_2 - \omega_1 = \alpha t$$

$$\omega_2 = \frac{d\theta}{dt} = \omega_1 + \alpha t$$

$$\Delta\theta = \int_1^2 \omega_1\, dt + \int_1^2 \alpha t\, dt$$

$$= \omega_1 t + \tfrac{1}{2}\alpha t^2.$$

PROBLEMS

1. Which of the following statements is *false*?

   a. A change in velocity is proportional to acceleration to the $\frac{1}{2}$ power.
   b. Acceleration is the second derivative of displacement with respect to time.
   c. Angular displacement is proportional to angular velocity and angular acceleration.
   d. Angular velocity is proportional to the product of acceleration and displacement to the 2nd power.
   e. Angular velocity is proportional to the first derivative of angular displacement.

2. The angular speed of a wheel changes from 3 rps to 12 rps in 2 seconds. What is the number of revolutions made in 2 seconds?

   a. 16
   b. 24
   c. 72
   d. 100
   e. 125

Check your answers.

Answers

1. d.
2. a.

C. RELATIVE KINEMATICS

Absolute kinematics is based on motion relative to some fixed point such as the earth. For example, displacement is thought of in absolute terms in the statement, "ten miles from City A."

In mechanisms it is sometimes useful to consider motion of one point with respect to another when both are moving. Consider the wheel below which is rotating and moving linearly at the same time:

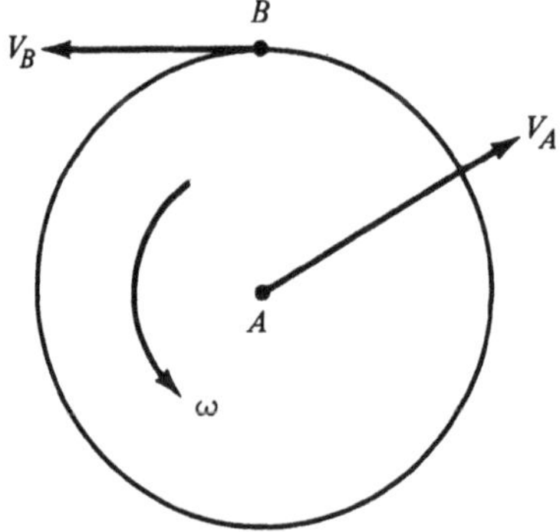

v_B is the tangential velocity of point B.

v_A is the linear velocity of point A.

A vector diagram of these two velocities with the absolute velocity added to complete a vector polygon is shown below:

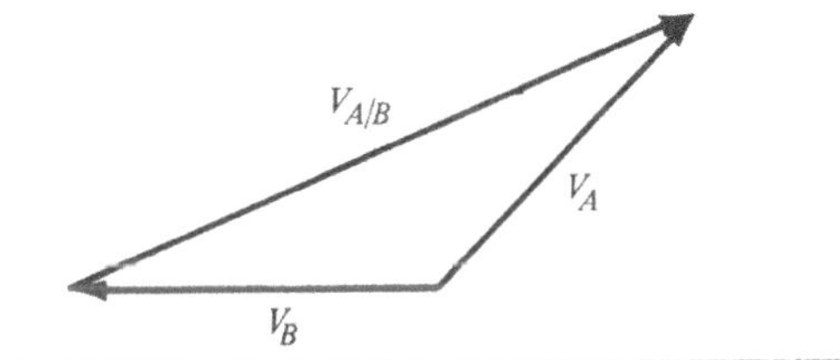

Note that v_A is the vector sum of v_B and $v_{A/B}$ (the relative velocity of A with respect to B). Therefore, v_A is

$$\vec{v}_A = \vec{v}_{A/B} + \vec{v}_B.$$

The same relationships hold for displacement and acceleration.

> Relative Displacement:
> $$\vec{s}_A = \vec{s}_{A/B} + \vec{s}_B.$$
> Relative Velocity:
> $$\vec{v}_A = \vec{v}_{A/B} + \vec{v}_B.$$
> Relative Acceleration:
> $$\vec{a}_A = \vec{a}_{A/B} + \vec{a}_B.$$

Example

In the crank-slider mechanism shown below, what is the angular velocity of the 6″ connecting rod at the time when $\theta = 60°$?

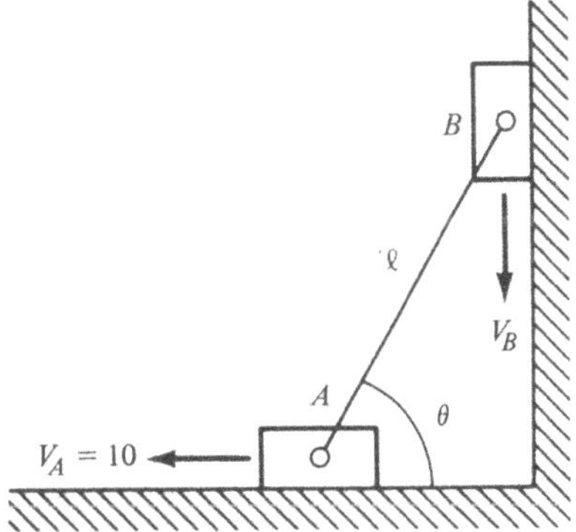

Note that $\vec{v}_{A/B}$ can only be perpendicular to the rigid link.

$$\vec{v}_A = \vec{v}_{A/B} + \vec{v}_B.$$

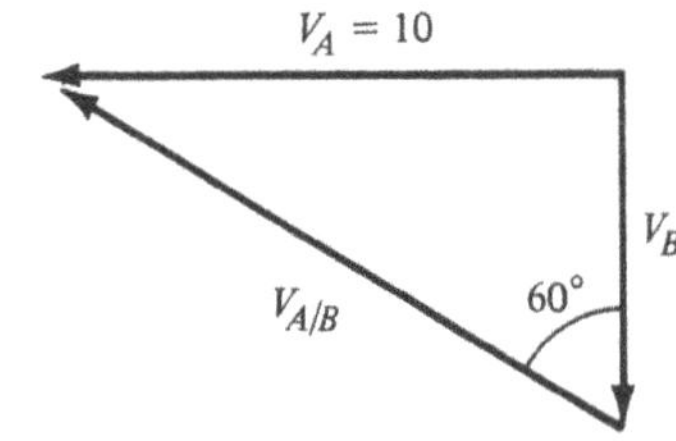

$$v_{A/B} = \frac{10}{\sin 60°} = 11.5 \text{ ft/sec.}$$

$$\omega = \frac{v_{A/B}}{\ell} = \frac{11.5}{\frac{1}{2}} = 23 \text{ rad/sec.}$$

PROBLEMS

1. The wheel shown below is rolling down a 30° incline. Point A and Point B are on the periphery.

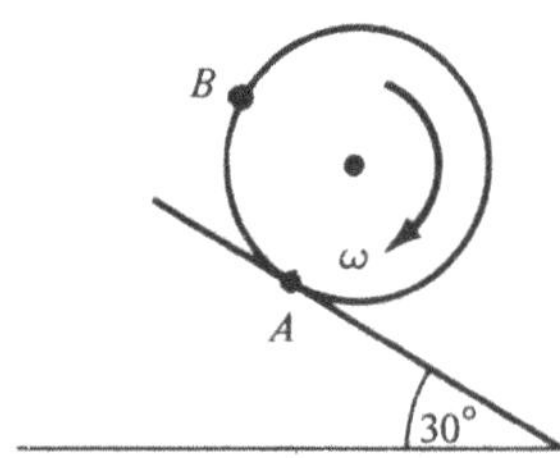

What is the direction of $v_{A/B}$?

a. 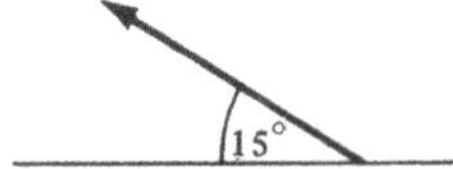

b. 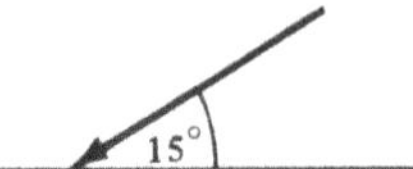

c. 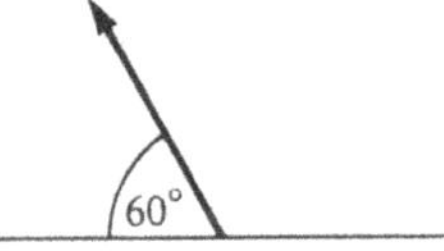

d. 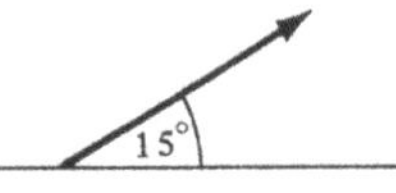

e.

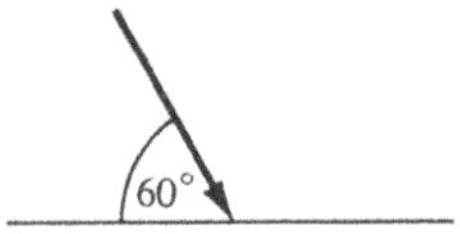

2. In the slider-crank shown below:

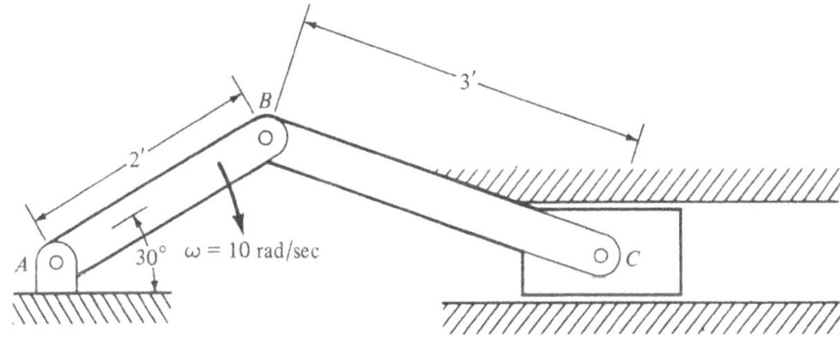

what is the velocity of C at the instant shown?

a. 20 ft/sec.
b. 23 ft/sec.
c. 17 ft/sec.
d. 52 ft/sec.
e. 40 ft/sec.

Check your answers.

Answers

1. b.
2. c.

D. VECTOR MULTIPLICATION

Vectors can be multiplied as well as added. Three different types of vector multiplication may be used.

1. Scalar Product

A vector multiplied by a scalar yields a vector:

$$\vec{A} = b\vec{C}$$

where $\vec{A}$ and $\vec{C}$ are vectors and b is a scalar.
Graphically:

C

A

$$\frac{|A|}{|C|} = b.$$

The vectors involved in a scalar product operation are along the same line of action.

2. Dot Product

A vector multiplied by a vector yields a scalar:

$$\vec{A} \cdot \vec{B} = c.$$

Graphically:

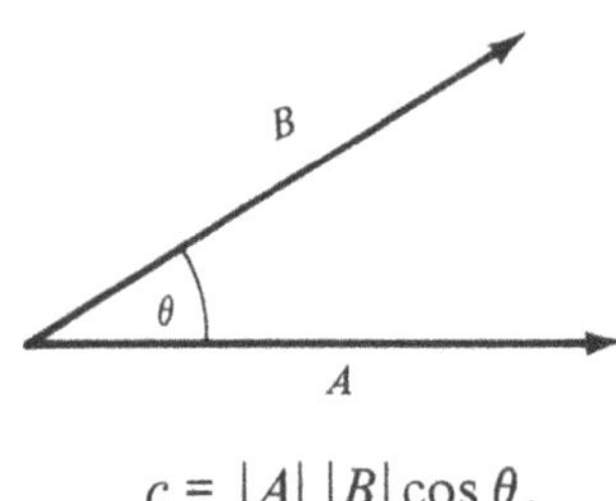

$$c = |A|\,|B| \cos \theta.$$

3. Cross Product

A vector times a vector yields a vector:

$$\vec{A} \times \vec{B} = \vec{C}.$$

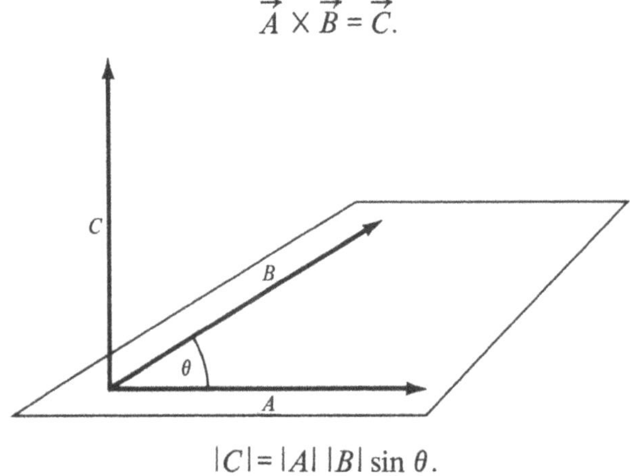

$$|C| = |A|\,|B| \sin \theta.$$

When the angle between A and B is 90°, $\sin \theta = 1$ and all vectors are mutually orthogonal.

> Scalar Product:
>
> $$\vec{A} = b\vec{C}.$$
>
> Dot Product:
>
> $$\vec{A} \cdot \vec{B} = c.$$
>
> Cross Product:
>
> $$\vec{A} \times \vec{B} = \vec{C}.$$

Example

The product of two vectors not equal to zero is zero. What operation is involved, and what is the orientation of these vectors with respect to each other?

The dot product operation

$$\vec{A} \cdot \vec{B} = c$$

yields

$$c = |A|\,|B| \cos \theta .$$

c equals zero when θ equals 90°. Hence, this is a dot product operation between two orthogonal vectors.

PROBLEM

To be completely analogous to velocity, rotational velocity ω must also be a vector. Given that

$$\vec{v} = \vec{r} \times \vec{\omega},$$

what is the vector direction of ω in the spinning wheel shown below?

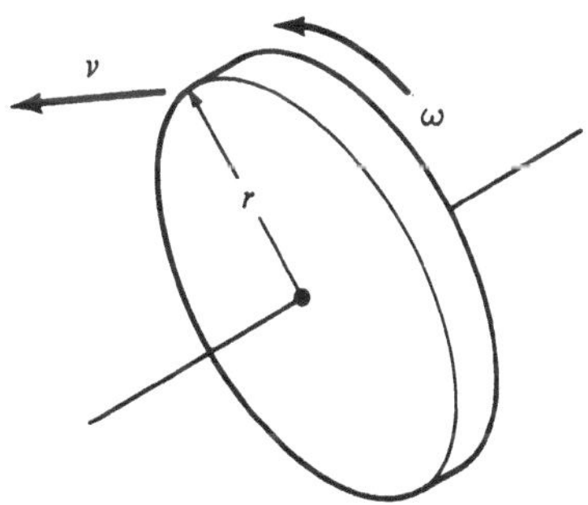

a. Tangential.
b. Radial.
c. Axial.
d. Vector sum of $\vec{v}$ and $\vec{r}$.
e. None of the above.

Check your answer.

Answer

c.

E. FORCES

If Newton's Law is differentiated with constant mass, the result is:

$$F = m\frac{dv}{dt}$$

or

$$F = ma.$$

In the conventional system of units,
F is in lb,
m is in slugs,
a is in ft/sec^2.
In the SI system (systeme international):
F is in Newtons,
m is in kilograms,
a is in meters/sec^2.
The magnitude of the unit "slug" is determined in the earth's gravitational field by weighing a mass. In this case, force due to gravity is weight, and one slug weighs 32.2 lb.

The rotational analogue of force is torque. Newton's Law becomes

$$\tau = I\alpha$$

in rotational terms, where
τ = torque in lb-ft,
I = moment of inertia slug-ft^2,
α = radial acceleration in rad/sec^2.

Newton's Law:
Linear:
$F = ma.$
Rotational:
$\tau = I\alpha.$

Example

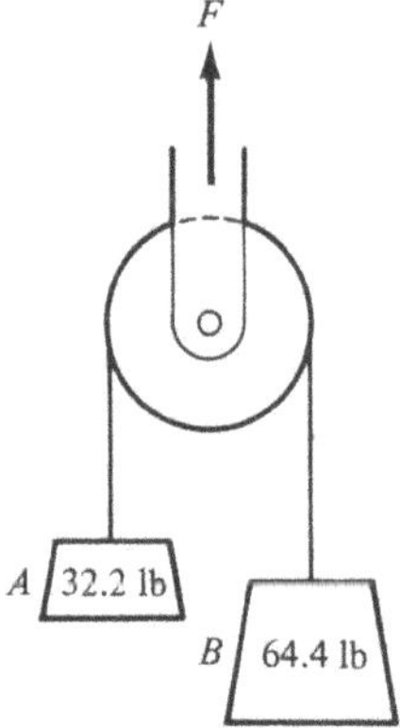

The acceleration of the two masses is as follows:
Net force, 32.2 lb down on body B;
Total mass, 3 slugs;

$$a = F/m = \frac{32.2}{3} = 10.7 \text{ ft/sec}^2.$$

Force on pully:
Force due to body A:

$$F = 32.2 + (1)(10.7) = 42.9 \text{ lb}.$$

Force due to body B

$$F = 64.4 - (2)(10.7) = 43.0 \text{ lb}.$$

Net force: 85.9 lb.

PROBLEMS

1. A V-belt drive on a 12-inch pully has a belt tension of 30 lb on the slack side and 60 lb on the tight side. What is the torque exerted on the pully?

   a. 90.
   b. 120.
   c. 15.
   d. 30.
   e. 20.

2. The maximum acceleration of an elevator whose cable strength is 2000 lb and whose load is 1000 lb is:

   a. 32.2 ft/sec^2.
   b. 2 ft/sec^2.
   c. 64.4 ft/sec^2.
   d. 4 ft/sec^2.
   e. None of the above.

Check your answers.

Answers

1. c.
2. a.

F. CENTRIFUGAL FORCE

Consider a wheel rotating at a constant angular velocity. A point on the periphery of the wheel has a tangential velocity that is constant in magnitude. But, as the point moves, the direction of the velocity vector changes. This change in direction is an acceleration, just as is a change in velocity magnitude.

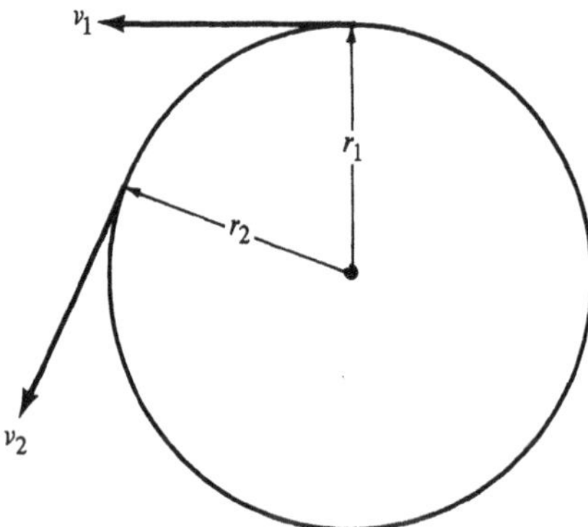

The wheel rotates through a small angle $d\theta$, causing a small change in direction of velocity, vector $\vec{v}$, from $t = 1$ to $t = 2$.
Vector diagram:

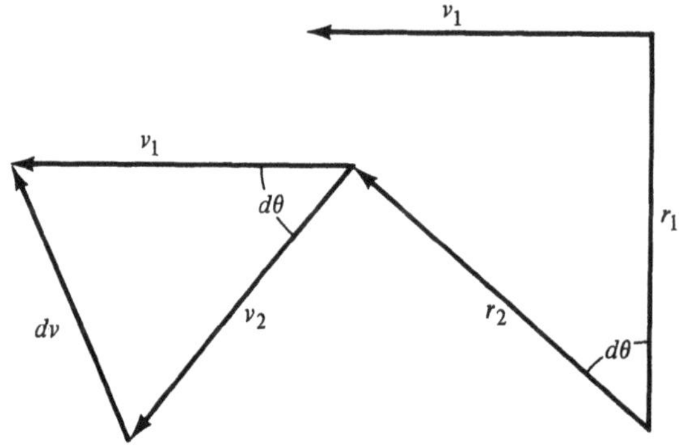

For small angles, for θ in radians,

$$dv = v \sin \theta \approx v\theta$$

$$dx = r \sin \theta \approx r\theta.$$

Radial acceleration due to this change in direction of the velocity vector is

$$a_R = \frac{dv}{dt} = \frac{v\theta}{dt} = \frac{v}{r}\frac{dx}{dt} = \frac{v^2}{r},$$

or, in terms of radial velocity,

$$a_R = r\omega^2.$$

This is the acceleration that causes centrifugal force.

Centrifugal Acceleration:

$$a = r\omega^2 \quad \text{or} \quad a = \frac{v^2}{r}.$$

Centrifugal Force:

$$F = mr\omega^2 \quad \text{or} \quad F = \frac{mv^2}{r}.$$

Direction: radial.

Example

A curve in the road with radius of curvature of 120 ft is banked so there is no reliance on friction with the road when a car is traveling at 30 ft/sec. What is the angle of the banked curve?

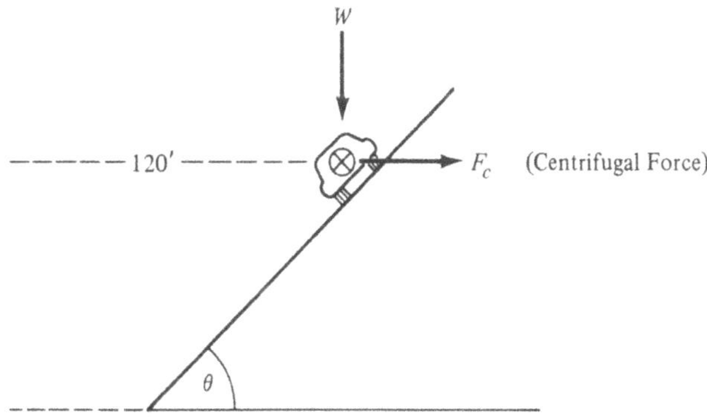

Force tending to cause the car to slip up the curve:

$$F_c \cos\theta.$$

Force tending to cause the car to slip down the curve:

$$W \sin\theta.$$

Equating these two forces:

$$W \sin\theta = \frac{W}{g}\,\frac{v^2}{r}\cos\theta$$

$$\tan\theta = \frac{v^2}{rg} = \frac{(30)^2}{(32)(120)} = 0.234$$

$$\theta = 13.2°.$$

PROBLEMS

1. A carnival loop-the-loop car weighs 850 pounds loaded. What must be its speed at the top of the 30 ft loop to keep it from falling?

   a. 22 ft/sec.
   b. 17 ft/sec.
   c. 28 ft/sec.
   d. 31 ft/sec.
   e. 8 ft/sec.

2. A train weighing 50 tons travels around a flat curve of 1000 ft radius at a speed of 45 mph. What is the nearest force on the rails?

   a. 218 tons.
   b. 187 tons.
   c. 7 tons.
   d. 5 tons.
   e. 3 tons.

Check your answers.

Answers

1. a.
2. c.

G. IMPULSE AND MOMENTUM

Differentiating Newton's Law with the product mv as an entity yields:

$$F = \frac{d(mv)}{dt}$$

$$F\,dt = d(mv)$$

$$F\,\Delta t = m_2 v_2 - m_1 v_1 .$$

The term on the left is called *impulse*—the product of force and time. The term on the right is a *change in momentum.*

In the absence of a force, we have

$$mv_{\text{initial}} = mv_{\text{final}}.$$

This is called *conservation of momentum.*

In a momentum conserving system, we deal with two types of collisions.

1. Elastic Collisions

Elastic collisions are like billiard balls where all the momentum of one ball is transferred to another. Consider the vector diagram of the billiard ball collision diagrammed below:

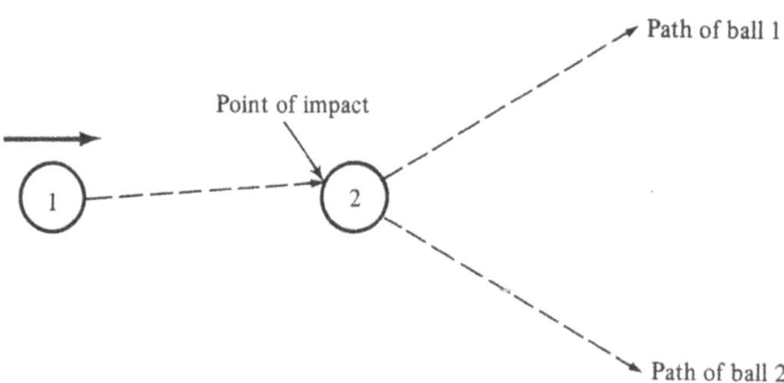

All the initial momentum of ball 1 is transferred to the x component of momentum in ball 1 and ball 2 after the collision. The y components of momentum for ball 1 and ball 2 are equal and opposite, so their sum is zero.

2. Sticking Collisions

Sticking collisions occur when two colliding objects stick together after a collision. A large rock falling into a moving gondola car is a sticking collision. The initial momentum is the mass of the car times its velocity. The final momentum is the mass of the car, plus rock, times its velocity.

Momentum, like all other kinematic and dynamic terms, has a rotational analogue. In rotational terms, the impulse–momentum law is

$$\tau t = \Delta(I\omega).$$

> Impulse-Momentum:
>
> $$F_t = \Delta(mv)$$
>
> $$\tau t = \Delta(I\omega).$$
>
> Conservation of Momentum:
>
> $$mv_{\text{initial}} = mv_{\text{final}}$$
>
> $$I\omega_{\text{initial}} = I\omega_{\text{final}}.$$

Example

A flywheel weighing 2000 lb has a radius of gyration of 4 feet. If there is a driving torque of 500 lb-ft and a resisting torque of 200 lb-ft, find the time required to increase its speed from 20 to 80 revolutions per minute.

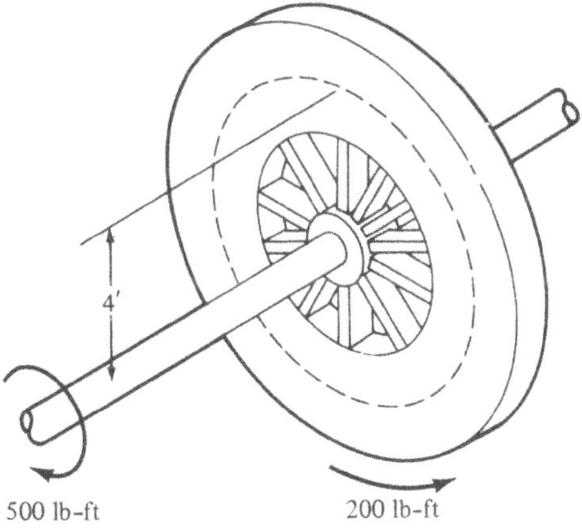

Change in angular velocity is given by

$$(80 - 20)\frac{2\pi}{60} = 6.28 \text{ rad/sec} = \Delta\omega.$$

Moment of inertia $I = mr^2$, where m is mass and r is radius of gyration:

$$I = mr^2 = \frac{W}{g} r^2 = \frac{2000}{32.2}(4)^2 = 994 \text{ ft-lb-sec}^2.$$

Solving by impulse–momentum for rotation:

$$\int_0^t \Sigma\tau \, dt = I\omega - I\omega_0.$$

For constant τ, the equation becomes

$$\Sigma\tau t = I(\omega - \omega_0).$$

Substituting the values given for this problem:

$$(500 - 200)t = 994(6.28)$$

$$t = \frac{994(6.28)}{300} = 20.8 \text{ sec.}$$

PROBLEMS

1. What is the recoil velocity of a wheeled cannon weighing 1000 lb and shooting a 30-lb ball at 900 ft/sec?

   a. 36 ft/sec.
   b. 18 ft/sec.
   c. 22 ft/sec.
   d. 27 ft/sec.
   e. None of these.

2. The same cannon fires into the wall of a fort. The cannon ball penetrates the fort wall in 0.1 seconds and exits at 100 ft/sec. What force was imparted to the wall of the fort?

   a. 135 tons.
   b. 120 tons.
   c. 3.8 tons.
   d. 7.6 tons.
   e. 88 tons.

Check your answers.

Answers

1. d.
2. c.

H. ENERGY

Energy is not a Newtonian quantity nor a vector; however, it involves the same kinematic quantities used in Newtonian physics when dealing with mechanically derived energy. *Mechanical energy* is defined as

$$E = Fx,$$

i.e., a force acting over a distance. If force is not constant but depends on distance, as in the case of a spring, then

$$E = \int F\,dx.$$

Three types of mechanical energy are considered here.

1. Friction Energy

Friction force is a constant, dependent on the nature of the friction surfaces and the normal force between them:

$$F_f = \mu N,$$

where μ is the coefficient of friction and N is the normal force. Frictional energy is

$$E = F_f x.$$

2. Potential Energy

Potential energy is the energy related to position in the earth's gravitational field. It is the amount of energy expended in raising an object or the amount of energy derived in lowering it. Since gravitational force (weight) equals mg,

$$E = \int mg\,dx = mgx = Wx,$$

i.e., energy equals the weight times the distance relative to the earth.

3. Kinetic Energy

Kinetic energy is the energy associated with velocity. Since

$$F = ma,$$

we have

$$\begin{aligned} E &= \int ma\,dx \\ &= \int m\frac{dv}{dt}\,dx \\ &= \int mv\,dv \\ &= \tfrac{1}{2}mv^2. \end{aligned}$$

Kinetic energy has a rotational analogue:

$$E = \tfrac{1}{2}I\omega^2.$$

When energy is converted from one of these three types to another, it is not lost; this is called *conservation of energy*.

Friction Energy:
$$FE = F_f x.$$
Potential Energy:
$$PE = Wx.$$
Kinetic Energy:
$$KE = \frac{1}{2} m v^2$$
$$KE = \frac{1}{2} I \omega^2.$$

Example

A 6-lb mall drives a spike 1″ into a board. The mall has an initial velocity of 15 ft/sec. What is the average force on the board?

The initial kinetic energy of the mall is dissipated in the board:

$$Fx = \frac{1}{2} m v^2$$

$$F = \frac{6}{32.2} \frac{(15)^2}{2} \frac{12}{1} = 251 \text{ lb.}$$

PROBLEMS

1. A linear spring is compressed from 6 in. to 4 in. The spring constant is 15 lb/in. How much energy was expended?

   a. 15 lb-in.
   b. 60 lb-in.
   c. 30 lb-in.
   d. 90 lb-in.
   e. 120 lb-in.

2. A 12-in.-diameter right circular cylinder rolls down a plane. The axis of the cylinder drops 4 ft. What is the linear velocity when the cylinder is rolling horizontally?

   a. 17 ft/sec.
   b. 13 ft/sec.
   c. 11 ft/sec.
   d. 22 ft/sec.
   e. 19 ft/sec.

Check your answers.

Answers

1. c.
2. b.

I. AFTERNOON PROBLEM SET

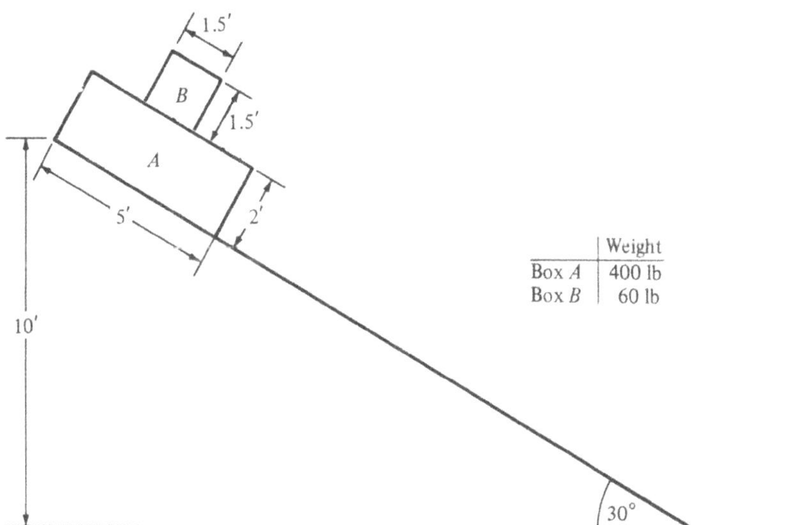

	Weight
Box *A*	400 lb
Box *B*	60 lb

1. The two boxes with uniform density slide down the frictionless plane. What is the velocity when they are first traveling horizontally?

   a. 16.1 ft/sec.
   b. 25.3 ft/sec.
   c. 21.9 ft/sec.
   d. 23.4 ft/sec.
   e. 10.8 ft/sec.

2. If the coefficient of friction on the plane is 0.3, what is the velocity when the front of the box is at the end of the plane?

   a. 15.2.
   b. 25.1.
   c. 16.4.
   d. 8.5.
   e. 14.7.

3. At what average rate is heat generated (Btu/hr) as the box goes down the plane?

   a. 276.
   b. 1.54.
   c. 4200.
   d. 12,500.
   e. 2,100.

4. In an attempt to overcome friction, 4 cylindrical wheels are added (negligible ground clearance) at each corner of *A*:

   Radius of gyration = 2 ft, Weight (total) = 50 lb.

   The final velocity when first horizontal now is nearest to:

   a. 45.
   b. 7.3.
   c. 16.
   d. 9.
   e. 23.

5. At the starting point, the coefficient of friction between A and B is at least:

a. 0.45.
b. 0.50.
c. 0.28.
d. 0.58.
e. 0.25.

6. Assume the boxes without wheels are traveling on the horizontal plane at 15 ft/sec. They pass over a 10-ft section where $\mu = 0.2$. How far does B move with respect to A if $\mu = 0.8$?

a. 4.4 ft.
b. 0 ft.
c. 2.5 ft.
d. 0.66 ft.
e. 13.2 ft.

7. At the far end of the horizontal plane there is no friction. The boxes are traveling 10 ft/sec. Assume B is fastened to A, and the motion of A is retarded by a spring, $K = 50$ lb/in. What is the maximum spring deflection?

a. 3 in.
b. 1.5 ft.
c. 2.3 ft.
d. 13 in.
e. 5.2 ft.

8. Consider the system consisting of blocks A and B resting on the horizontal frictionless plane. Block B is in the center of block A. A force is applied to block A that results in block B moving to the position shown below:

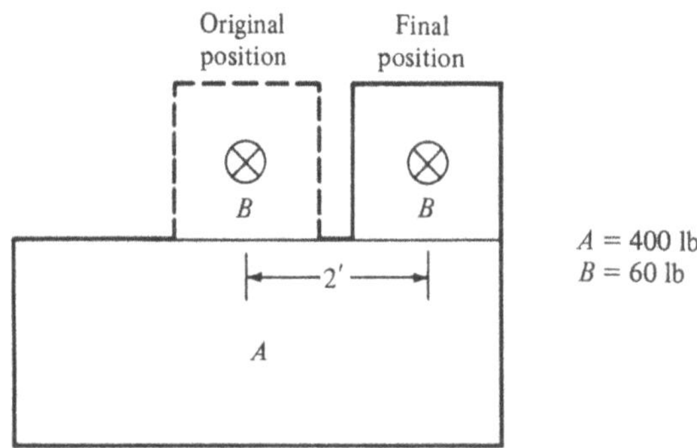

This reaction happened in 1 sec, during which time block A moved 8 ft. What force was required?

a. 210 lb.
b. 206 lb.
c. 221 lb.
d. 213 lb.
e. 229 lb.

9. What is the coefficient of friction between A and B?

a. 0.125.
b. 0.250.
c. 0.375.
d. 0.500.
e. 0.625.

10. What is the velocity of B at the final position?

    a. 14 ft/sec.
    b. 12 ft/sec.
    c. 8 ft/sec.
    d. 6 ft/sec.
    e. 4 ft/sec.

Check your answers.

Answers

1. d.
2. a.
3. c.
4. e.
5. d.
6. b.
7. b.
8. b.
9. a.
10. e.

16 Mechanics of Materials

Discussion of and problems related to Hook's Law and deformation, Poisson's Ratio, thermal expansion, pipes and pressure vessels, rivet joints, shafts, stresses in beams, deflection of beams, and columns.

A. INTRODUCTION

The fundamental concept in mechanics of materials is stress—the distribution of external forces within a material. Stress is similar to pressure and is defined the same way, as a force divided by area. It differs from pressure, however, in that it has directionality and nonuniformity. This is due to the fact that stress relates to solids whereas pressure relates to fluids.

The simplest kind of stress results when a prism is loaded *axially* with a load *normal* to a face.

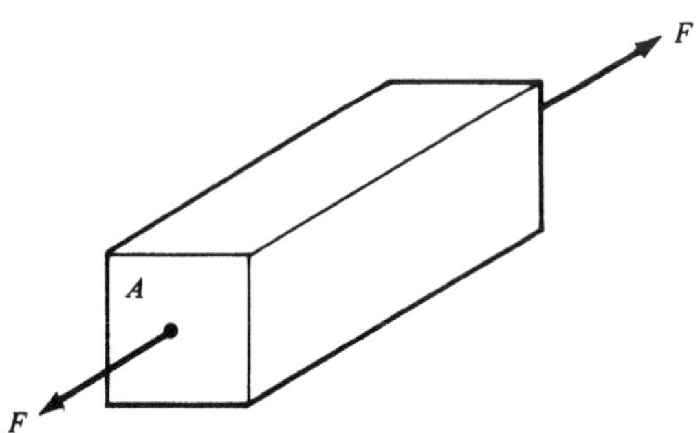

The resulting stress is a *tensile stress*:

$$S_t = \frac{F_{\text{normal}}}{A_{\text{normal}}}.$$

Because of the axial loading, it is uniform throughout the prism.

Compressive stress is similarly defined with the forces reversed.

Shearing stress results if we examine a plane within the body that is not normal to the axis:

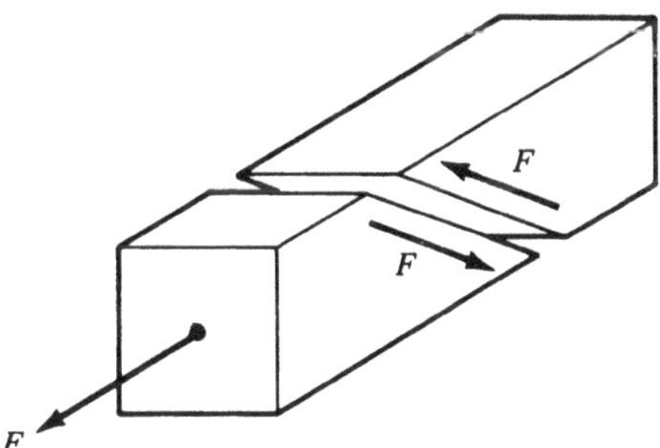

The forces will be resisted at the plane shown by a shearing stress which is defined as the force *parallel* to the shearing plane, divided by the area:

$$S_s = \frac{F_{\text{parallel}}}{A_{\text{shear}}}.$$

An axially loaded body is one in which the load is centroidal and the unit stresses are uniformly distributed across the cross section at any point. If the load is not axial, then the stress is nonuniform.

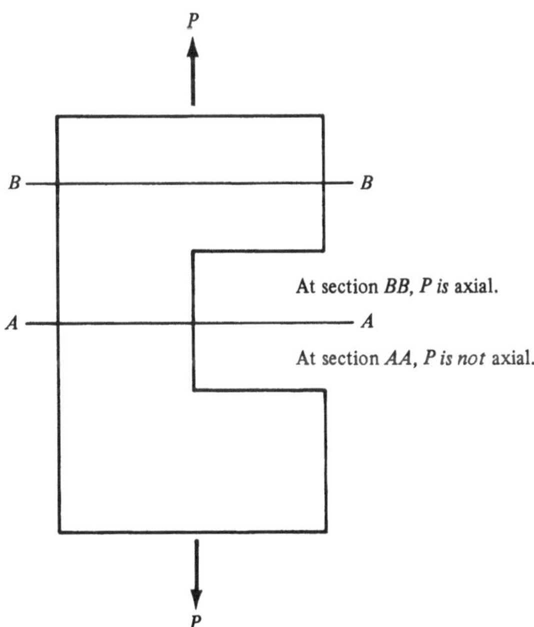

If the load is not a centroidal load, the member can be said to be eccentrically loaded.

Special cases of nonuniform stresses will be covered in later sections.

Stress:	
Tensile:	$S = F/A$.
Compressive:	$S = F/A$.
Shear:	$S = F/A$.

Example

The best concrete available has an allowable stress of 5000 psi. What is the minimum diameter permissible on the support shown below to support a twenty ton load?

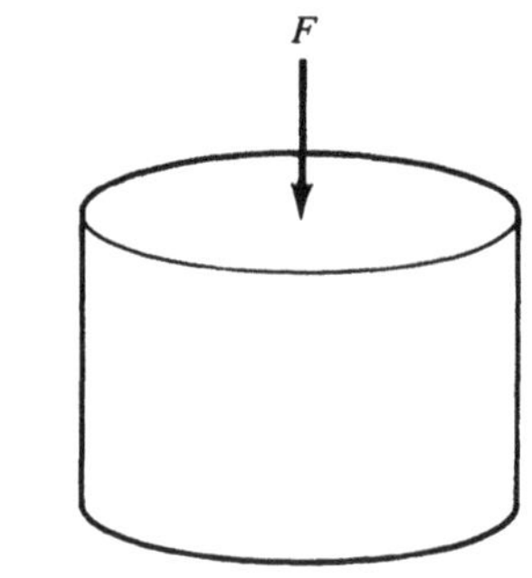

$$S = F/A$$

$$5000 = \frac{(20)(2000)}{\pi D^2/4}$$

$$D = \sqrt{\frac{40{,}000}{5{,}000} \cdot \frac{4}{\pi}} = 3.19 \text{ in.}$$

PROBLEMS

1. Which of the statements below is not correct?

   a. Eccentric loading produces nonuniform stress.
   b. Stress is directly proportional to force.
   c. In an axially loaded member, shearing stress is zero in a plane normal to the axis.
   d. Shearing stress is inversely proportional to the area normal to the force.
   e. Compressive stress in a normal plane is uniform if the force is axial.

2. What is the shearing stress in the $\frac{1}{2}$-in. pin illustrated below?

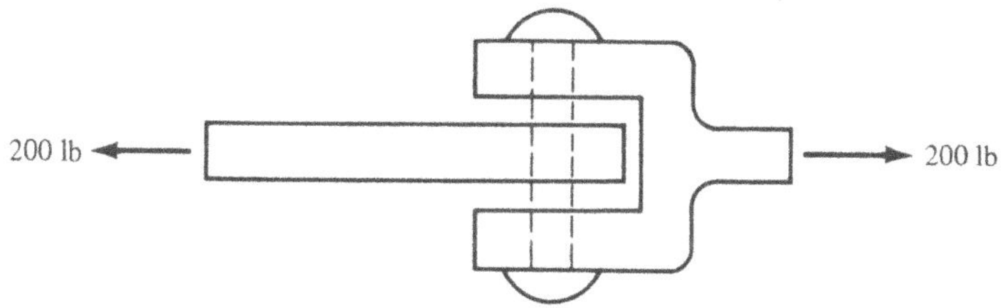

a. 1020 psi.
b. 258 psi.
c. 510 psi.
d. 2040 psi.
e. None of the above.

Check your answers.

Answers

1. d.
2. c. Shear occurs in two planes.

B. HOOK'S LAW AND DEFORMATION

Hook's Law states that stress is proportional to strain, where strain is defined as *unit* deformation. In other words, in the stress region where Hook's Law applies the stress–strain curve is linear.

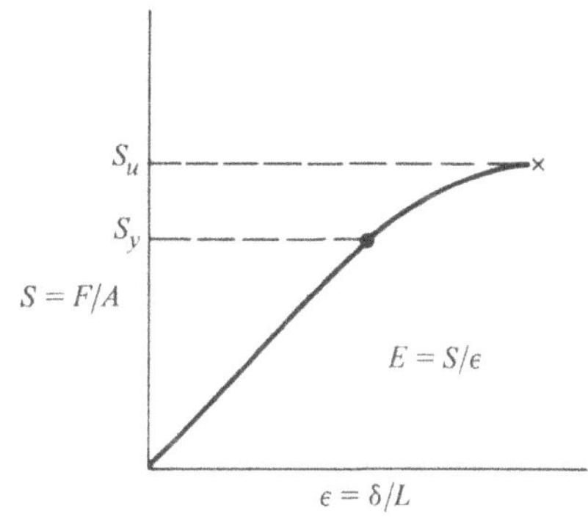

In the linear region the slope of the curve E is a property of the material called the *modulus of elasticity* or *Young's modulus.*

In the linear region deformation is called *elastic deformation* because the material does not take a permanent set. In this region the material behaves exactly like a spring; the modulus of elasticity is analogous to the spring constant. At stress level S_y the curve becomes nonlinear. This is called the *yield point* and deformation at these stress levels is plastic (permanent set occurs). At stress level S_u the material fails. This is called *ultimate stress.*

> Stress vs. Strain:
>
> $$S/\epsilon = E(\text{psi}),$$
>
> where
>
> $$S = F/A\,(\text{psi})$$
>
> $$\epsilon = \delta/L\,(\text{in./in.})$$

Example

A 1-in. cube compresses 0.001 in. under a 200 lb load. What is the modulus of elasticity?

Stress:

$$S = \frac{200}{1} = 200 \text{ psi.}$$

Strain:

$$\epsilon = \frac{0.001}{1} = 0.001$$

$$E = \frac{S}{\epsilon} = \frac{200}{0.001} = 200{,}000 \text{ psi.}$$

PROBLEMS

1. The Hook's-Law region of the stress–strain curve is:

   a. The area of plastic deformation.
   b. Reversible.
   c. Between yield and ultimate stress.
   d. The area where Young's modulus is proportional to stress to the $\frac{1}{2}$ power.
   e. A poor area to design to.

2. What amount of stretch would you expect in a 3-ft steel rod with a $\frac{1}{2}$-in. diameter loaded with a 500 lb weight? ($E = 30 \times 10^6$ psi.)

   a. 3.0×10^{-3} in.
   b. 2.5×10^{-4} in.
   c. 8.5×10^{-5} in.
   d. 7.5×10^{-4} in.
   e. 1.3×10^{-3} in.

Check your answers.

Answers

1. b.
2. a.

C. POISSON'S RATIO

When strain occurs in the axis of force application, a corresponding strain also occurs in the lateral dimension. For example, if a bar under tension elongates, it will become thinner. The ratio of these two strains is called *Poisson's Ratio*.

> Poisson's Ratio:
>
> $$\mu = \frac{\epsilon_{\text{lateral}}}{\epsilon_{\text{longitudinal}}}.$$
>
> Poisson's ratio is a property of the material.

Example

In the previous example of the 1-in. cube, if Poisson's Ratio is 0.33,

$$\epsilon_{\text{lateral}} = (0.33)\epsilon_{\text{longitudinal}}$$

$$= \frac{(0.33)(0.001)}{1} = 33 \times 10^{-5} \text{ in./in.}$$

Lateral deformation is

$$\delta_{\text{lateral}} = (33 \times 10^{-5})(1) = 33 \times 10^{-5} \text{ in.}$$

PROBLEM

A 4-in.-diameter steel shaft is under an axial compressive load of 100,000 psi. What is the minimum bearing size for this shaft? ($\mu = 0.3$)

a. 4.008 in.
b. 4.0002 in.
c. 4.003 in.
d. 4.0001 in.
e. 4.004 in.

Check your answer.

Answer

e.

D. THERMAL EXPANSION

When the temperature of most materials is increased, the material expands:

$$\delta_T = \alpha L \, \Delta T,$$

where α is called the coefficient of thermal expansion. Dividing by the length of the element yields thermal strain. No stress is induced in a member by temperature change unless the member is restrained from deforming.

Thermal Expansion:
$\delta_T = \alpha L\ \Delta T.$

Example

A concrete member 5 ft long is heated 100°F:

$$E = 2.5 \times 10^6 \text{ psi}$$

$$\alpha = 6.2 \times 10^{-6}(°\text{F})^{-1}$$

What is the increase in length if the member is free to move?

$$\begin{aligned}\delta &= L\alpha(\Delta T)\\ &= 5(6.2 \times 10^{-6})(100)\\ &= 3.1 \times 10^{-3} \text{ ft.}\end{aligned}$$

What stresses are induced if the member is restrained?

$$\begin{aligned}S &= E\epsilon = E\delta/L\\ &= (2.5 \times 10^6)\,\frac{(3.1 \times 10^{-3})}{5}\\ &= 1550 \text{ psi.}\end{aligned}$$

PROBLEM

An aluminum tube with a copper insert is restrained by two surfaces. What force is exerted on the surfaces by a 50°F temperature rise?

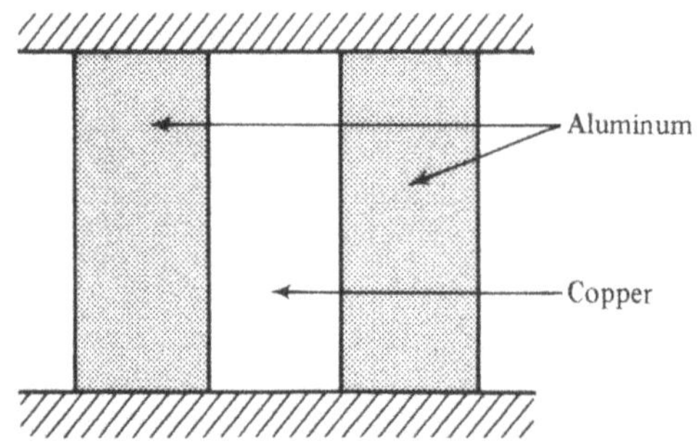

	Aluminum	*Copper*
area	12 in.^{2}	9 in.^{2}
Young's Modulus	10×10^6	16×10^6
Thermal expansion	25.7×10^{-6}	9.8×10^{-6}

a. 141,100 lb.
b. 224,760 lb.
c. 25,000 lb.
d. 11,700 lb.
e. 98,500 lb.

Check your answer.

Answer

b.

E. PIPES AND PRESSURE VESSELS

Hoop stress is the circumferential stress in a pipe or pressure vessel that is due to internal pressure. Longitudinal stress applies to cylindrical vessels in the longitudinal direction. The derivations follow the method below:

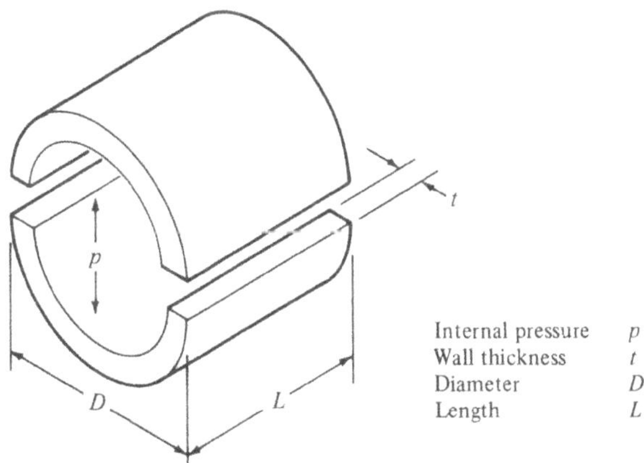

Force separating the two halves due to pressure:

$$F = pA = pD \qquad \text{(for unit length).}$$

This is opposed by the stress in the material:

$$F = SA = S2t \qquad \text{(for unit length).}$$

Therefore,

$$S = \frac{pD}{2t}.$$

Stress in Thin-walled Pipes and Pressure Vessels
(e.g., shrink fits and stresses in vertical water tanks):

Hoop tension or circumferential stress (pipe or vessel):

$$S_T = \frac{pD}{2t}.$$

Longitudinal stress (vessel):

$$S_L = \frac{pD}{4t}.$$

Spherical pressure vessel:

$$S = \frac{pD}{4t}.$$

p = unit stress due to fluid pressure (psi),
D = diameter of vessel (inside) (in.),
t = shell thickness (in.).

Example

A 12-in. pipe has a pressure head of 20 ft of water. What wall thickness is required if the ultimate stress level is 30 ksi?

$$t = \frac{pD}{2S} = \frac{(20)(62.4)(12)}{(144)(2)(30 \times 10^3)}$$

$$= 0.0017 \text{ in.}$$

PROBLEM

The steel cylindrical tank shown below has a wall thickness of 0.125 in. What is the maximum pressure permitted? (Allowable stress is 20 ksi.)

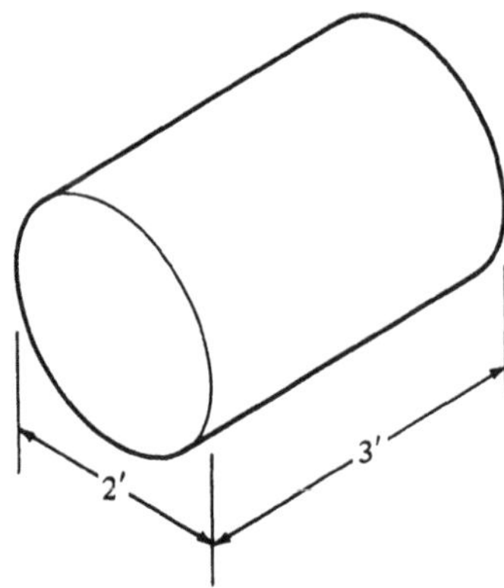

a. 625 psi.
b. 208 psi.
c. 1250 psi.
d. 416 psi.
e. 104 psi.

Check your answer.

Answer

b.

F. RIVET JOINTS

Rivets are commonly used to form joints in structural members and in pressure vessels. The method of analysis consists of finding the repeating pattern of the rivets and then analyzing that part of the joint. For example, if the rivets are spaced in a single line on 4-in. centers, a 4-in. sample of the joint will be representative of the total joint.

The ability of rivets to withstand forces is based on three important modes.

1. Single Shear

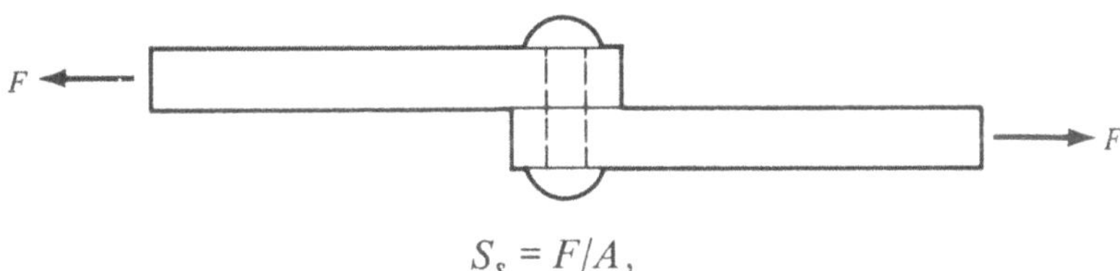

$$S_s = F/A,$$

where S_s is the allowable shear strength of the rivet material and A is the cross-sectional area of the rivet.

2. Shear of Base Material

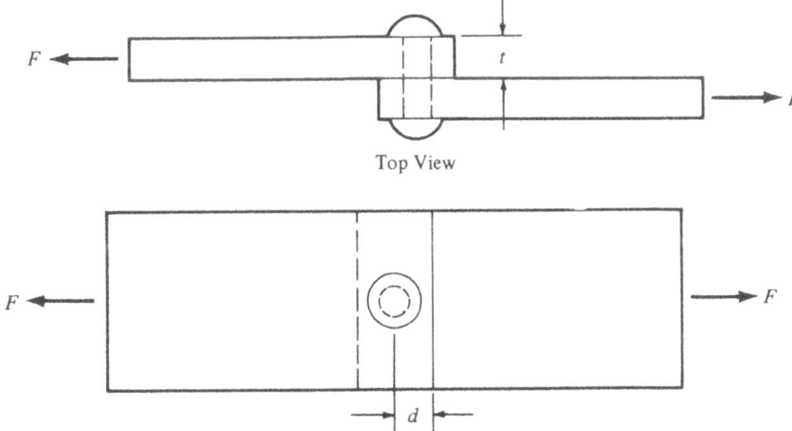

where S_s is the allowable shearing stress of the base material, t is the thickness of the base material, and d is the distance from the rivet to the edge.

3. Bearing

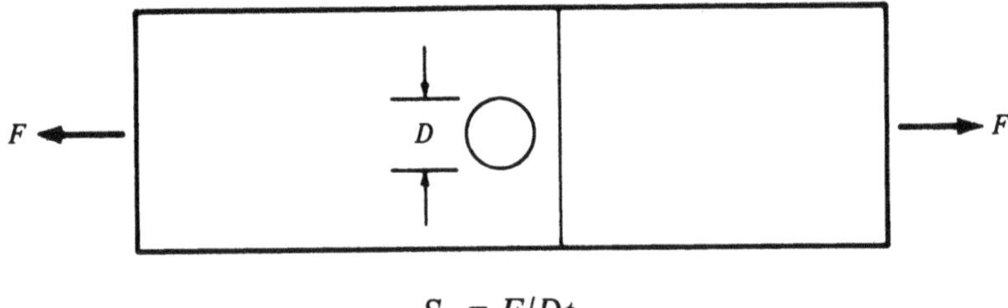

$$S_c = F/Dt,$$

where S_c is the allowable compressive stress of the base material, D is the diameter of the rivet, and t is the thickness of the base material.

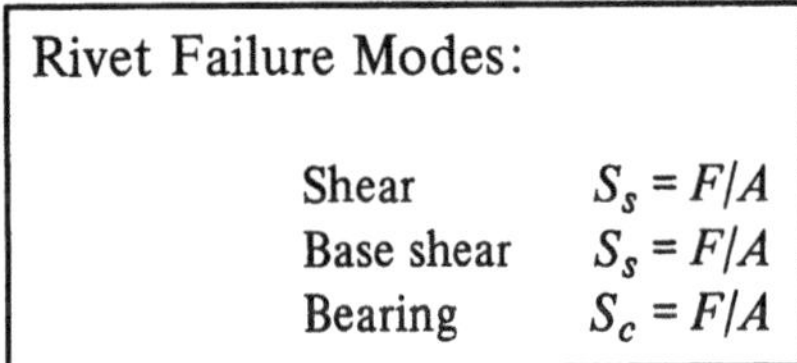

Rivet Failure Modes:

Shear	$S_s = F/A$
Base shear	$S_s = F/A$
Bearing	$S_c = F/A$

Example

At what force will the rivet joint shown below fail?

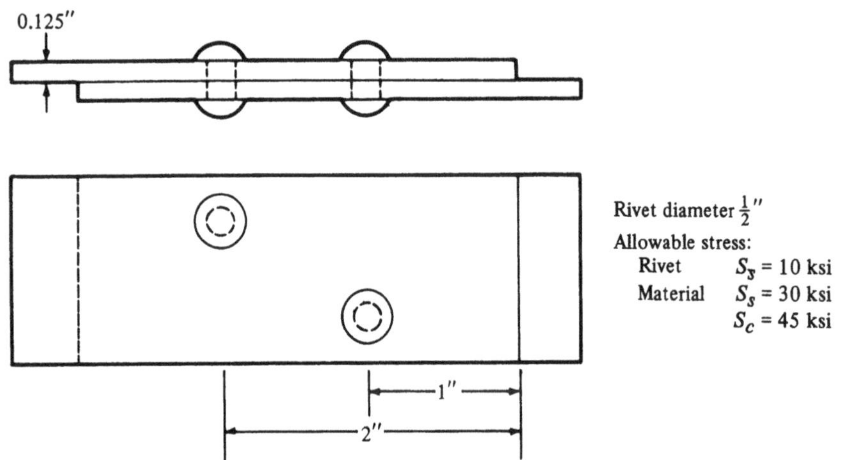

Rivet shear is

$$F = S_s A = (10 \times 10^3)(0.196)(2) = 3{,}920 \text{ lb.}$$

Material shear is

$$F = (2)(S_s)(2)(t)(d) = (30 \times 10^3)(2)(0.125) = 15{,}000 \text{ lb.}$$

Bearing force is

$$F = 2S_c Dt = (2)(45 \times 10^3)(0.5)(0.125) = 5{,}625 \text{ lb.}$$

Hence the rivets will fail in shear at a load of 3920 lb.

PROBLEM

A 6-in. ID pipe is made of $\frac{1}{8}$-in. steel plate fastened by a single row of $\frac{3}{8}$-in. diameter rivets spaced 4 in. apart. End distance is 1 in. Allowable stresses are as follows: shear, 12,000 psi; tension and compression, 19,000 psi. What hydraulic pressure is allowable?

a. 37.1 psi.
b. 1324 psi.
c. 55.0 psi.
d. 891 psi.
e. 243 psi.

Check your answer.

Answer

a. Bearing stress governs.

G. SHAFTS

Shafts resisting a torque are in shear. The stress profile of a solid circular shaft is shown below:

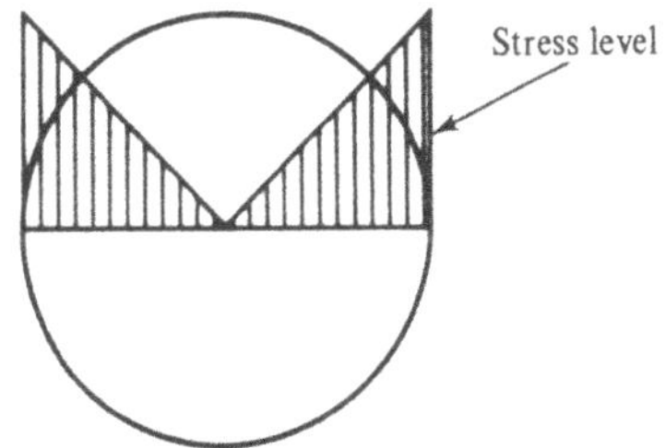

The stress is a maximum at the outer surface and is zero at the center.

Deflection of a shaft is described as its angle of twist θ.

Stress and Strain in Simple Torsion

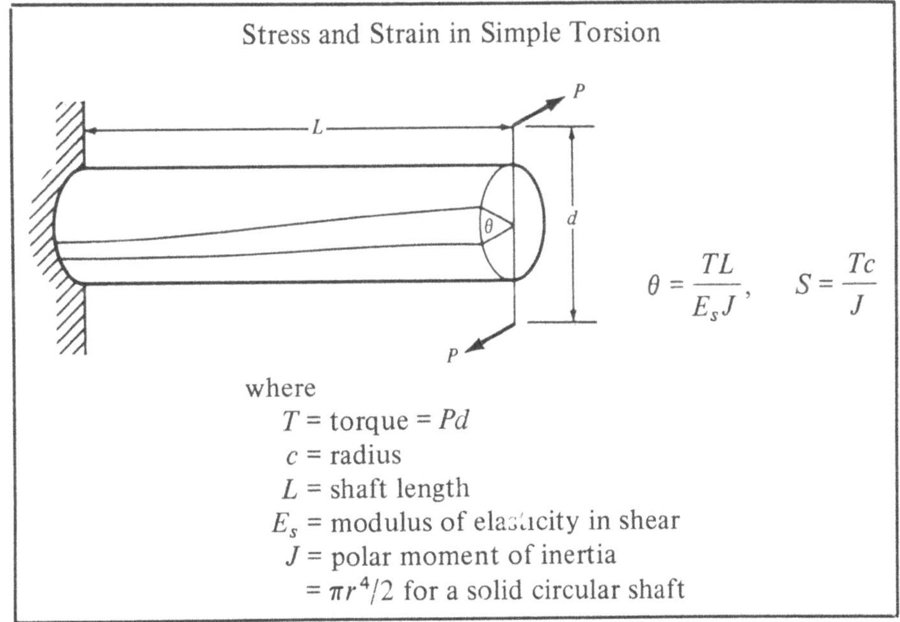

$$\theta = \frac{TL}{E_s J}, \quad S = \frac{Tc}{J}$$

where

T = torque = Pd
c = radius
L = shaft length
E_s = modulus of elasticity in shear
J = polar moment of inertia
= $\pi r^4/2$ for a solid circular shaft

Example

A 3 ft pully is driving a $1\frac{1}{2}$-in. circular shaft. Belt tensions are 500 and 200 lb. What deflection of the shaft occurs if its length is 48 in. and its shear modulus is 15×10^6 psi?

$$J = \frac{\pi(1.5)^4}{32} = 0.49 \text{ in.}^4$$

$$\theta = \frac{TL}{E_s J} = \frac{18(300)(48)}{(15 \times 10^6)(0.49)} = 3.53 \times 10^{-2} \text{ radians}$$

PROBLEMS

1. If the shaft of the preceding example is rotating at 200 rpm, what horsepower is transmitted?

   a. 10 hp.
   b. 12 hp.
   c. 15 hp.
   d. 17 hp.
   e. 19 hp.

2. What is the maximum stress in the shaft if it is a hollow shaft with ID = 1″?

   a. 10,400 psi.
   b. 9,800 psi.
   c. 7,600 psi.
   d. 12,700 psi.
   e. 16,300 psi.

Check your answers.

Answers

1. d.
2. a.

H. STRESSES IN BEAMS

The stresses in a beam are tensile or compressive. Since the beam flexes, these stresses are called *flexural stresses*. Consider a simply supported beam:

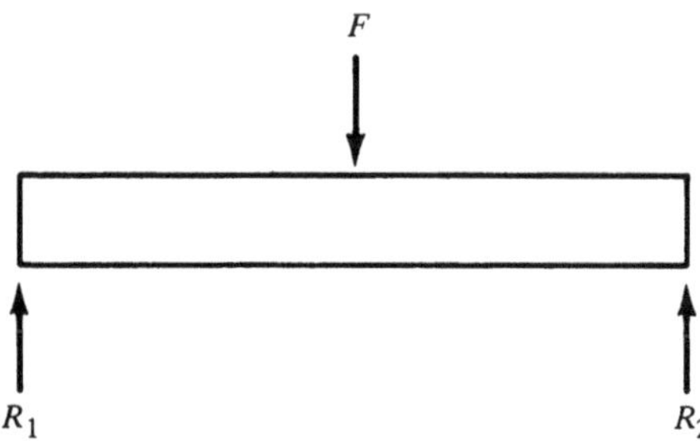

The moment in the beam is

$$M = Rx$$

where x is the distance from the end of the beam. The flexural stress depends on the moment:

$$S_f = \frac{Mc}{I}$$

where
M is the moment in the beam,
I is the moment of inertia of the cross-sectional area, and
c is the distance from the neutral axis.
The neutral axis is an axis passing through the centroid of the cross-sectional area of the beam.

Given a cross-sectional area, beam analysis consists of determining the maximum moment in a beam.

Shear and Moment Diagrams

Shear force in a beam is a measure of resistance to sliding on some given plane normal to the longitudinal axis of the beam. For example:

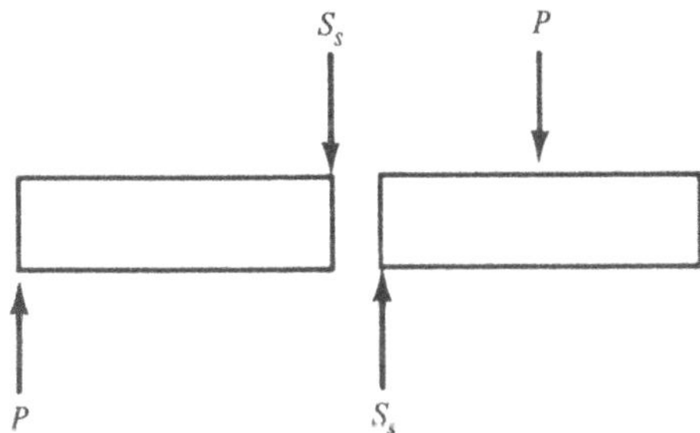

Shear may be defined as follows: The shear at any point in a beam is equal to the sum of all transverse loads acting to the left or right of a section.

The moment in a beam is maximum at the point where shear force is zero.

Typical Shear and Moment Diagrams for Various Loading Conditions

Concentrated Loads:

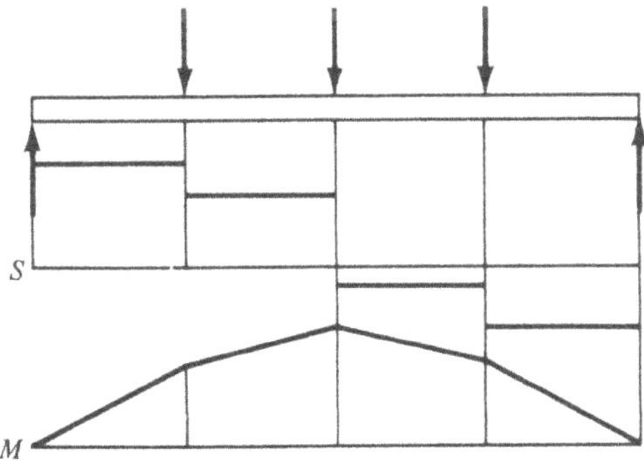

Bending moment M is the sum of all moments acting to the left or right of a section.
Uniformly Distributed Loads:

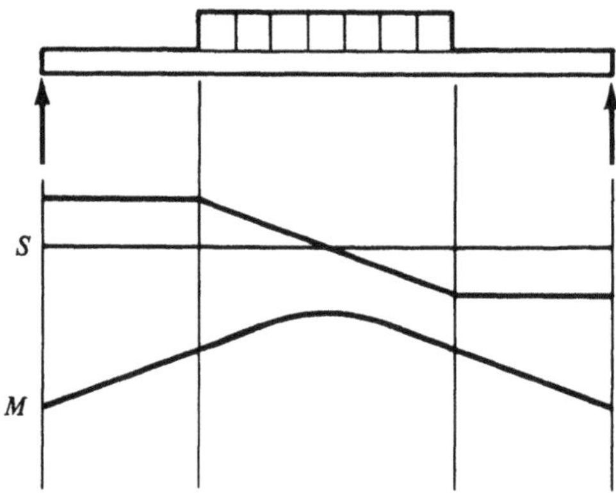

Uniformly Varying Loads:

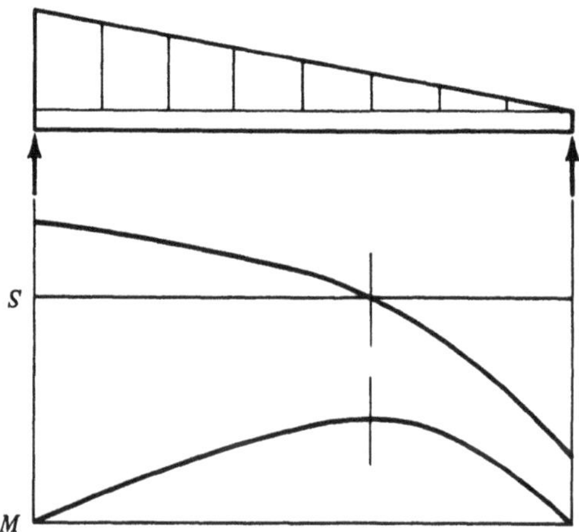

Beam Stress:

$$S_f = \frac{Mc}{I},$$

where
M = moment,
c = distance from neutral axis, and
I = cross-sectional area moment of inertia.
The moment in a beam is maximum where the shearing force is zero.

Example

Given a 30-ft simply supported beam of 6″ square cross section with a uniform load of 50 lb/ft, what is the maximum flexural stress?

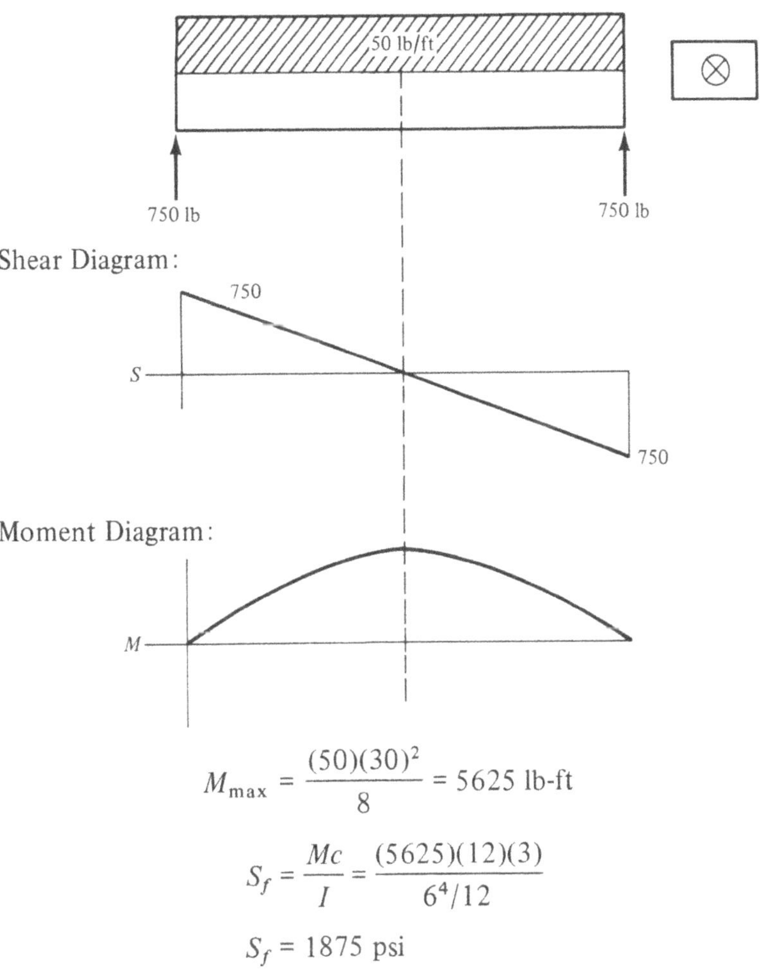

$$M_{\max} = \frac{(50)(30)^2}{8} = 5625 \text{ lb-ft}$$

$$S_f = \frac{Mc}{I} = \frac{(5625)(12)(3)}{6^4/12}$$

$$S_f = 1875 \text{ psi}$$

PROBLEMS

1. What is the maximum moment on a cantilevered beam 20 ft long with a 2000 lb load at the free end?

   a. 10,000 lb-ft.
   b. 20,000 lb-ft.
   c. 30,000 lb-ft.
   d. 40,000 lb-ft.
   e. 50,000 lb-ft.

2. If the beam above has a circular cross section, radius 6″, what is the maximum flexural stress?

   a. 2829 psi.
   b. 707 psi.
   c. 354 psi.
   d. 2264 psi.
   e. 968 psi.

Check your answers.

Answers

1. d.
2. a.

I. DEFLECTION OF BEAMS

The deflection of the beam at any given point is also of interest. From $dM = S\,dx$ we know that

$$\int_A^B dM = \int_A^B S\,dx.$$

This tells us that the change in moment between any two points A and B in a loaded beam is equal to the net area of the shear diagram between the two points. This says that the $dM/dx = S$ slope of the moment curve at any point in a loaded beam is numerically equal to the shear in the beam at that point. This relationship tells us that where the shear diagram passes through a zero value, the moment curve will be a maximum or minimum at that point, i.e., the slope of the moment curve will be zero at this point.

Beam Deflection—Double Integration Method

$$\frac{EI\,d^2y}{dx^2} = M,$$

where M is the bending moment at any point in a beam. Integrating the above once gives a general expression for the slope in a beam:

$$EI\frac{dy}{dx} = \text{slope} \times EI.$$

A second integration gives a general equation for the elastic curve of a beam:

$$EIy = \text{vertical displacement} \times EI.$$

NOTE: The equations for most common beams are available in handbooks.

Deflection of a Beam:

$$y = \int \frac{Mx}{EI}\,dx.$$

Example

What is the maximum deflection at the left load in the beam below?

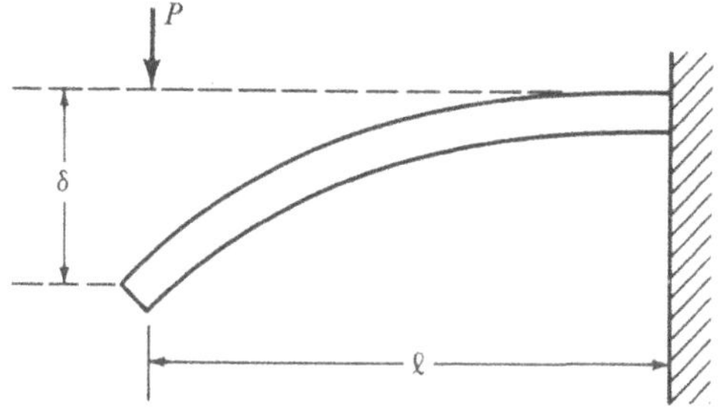

$$M = \frac{EI\, d^2y}{dx^2} = -P(\ell - x).$$

Integrating,

$$EI\frac{dy}{dx} = -\int (P\ell - Px)\, dx$$

$$= -P\ell x + \tfrac{1}{2}Px^2 + C_1.$$

when $x = 0$, $dy/dx = 0$, so $C_1 = 0$. Integrate again:

$$EIy = -\int (P\ell x + \tfrac{1}{2}Px^2)\, dx$$

$$= -\tfrac{1}{2}P\ell x^2 + \frac{Px^3}{6} + C_2.$$

When $y = 0$, $x = 0$, so $C_2 = 0$.

$$y = \frac{(Px^3/6) - (P\ell x^2/2)}{EI}.$$

PROBLEMS

1. The deflection at midspan of the uniformly loaded beam shown below is:

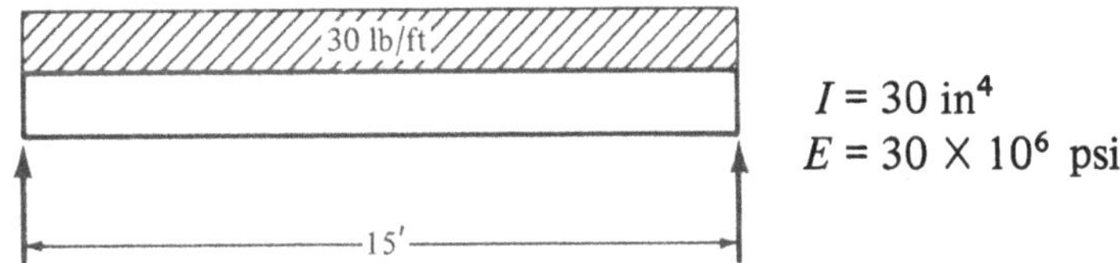

$I = 30$ in^4
$E = 30 \times 10^6$ psi

a. 0.0002 in.
b. 0.0020 in.
c. 0.038 in.
d. 0.0040 in.
e. 0.015 in.

2. The deflection of a simple beam is NOT:

a. Inversely proportional to the height of the beam to the fourth power.
b. Proportional to the length from the supports.

c. Proportional to the slope of the stress–strain curve for the material.
d. Inversely proportional to the area moment of inertia.
e. Proportional to the second integral of the radius of curvature.

Check your answers.

Answers

1. c.
2. c.

J. COLUMNS

Columns do not fail in compression as do compressively loaded prismatic members. They fail by buckling. Early experiments by Euler found that failure by buckling occurred when

$$\frac{\ell}{k} > 200,$$

where
ℓ is the length of the member, and
k is the least cross-sectional radius of gyration.
This, then, is the definition of a column.

Euler determined a critical axial force which would cause buckling for various end conditions.

Euler Equation for Columns:

Round-ended column:

$$P_{cr} = \frac{\pi^2 EI}{\ell^2}.$$

Fixed ends:

$$P_{cr} = \frac{4\pi^2 EI}{\ell^2}.$$

One end free, one end fixed:

$$P_{cr} = \frac{\pi^2 EI}{4\ell^2}.$$

P_{cr} = critical force that will cause buckling.

Example

A yardstick has cross-sectional dimensions of 3/16″ × 1″. What axial force will cause it to buckle?

Least radius of gyration:

$$K = \frac{3/16}{2\sqrt{3}} = 0.054$$

$$\frac{\ell}{K} = \frac{36}{0.054} = 666$$

Therefore, the yardstick is a column.

The modulus of elasticity of wood is $E = 1.5 \times 10^6$ psi. The moment of inertia of the yardstick is

$$I = \frac{(1)(3/16)^3}{12} = 5.49 \times 10^{-4} \text{ in.}^4$$

The critical force is, therefore,

$$P_{cr} = \frac{\pi^2 EI}{\ell^2} = 6.27 \text{ lb}$$

PROBLEMS

1. The slenderness ratio of a column is:

   a. Length divided by moment of inertia.
   b. Maximum radius of gyration divided by length.
   c. Moment of inertia times modulus of elasticity.
   d. Length divided by least radius of gyration.
   e. None of the above.

2. A 30-ft aluminum column made of a 3-ft, 2.31 lb/ft I-beam fixed at both ends has a critical force of:

   a. 558,700 lb.
   b. 1,551 lb.
   c. 387 lb.
   d. 223,484 lb.
   e. 968 lb.

Check your answers.

Answers

1. d.
2. b.

K. AFTERNOON PROBLEM SET

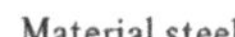

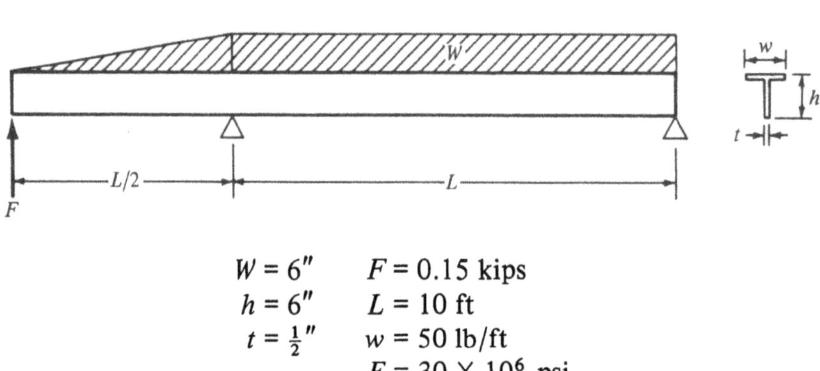

$W = 6''$ $\quad F = 0.15$ kips
$h = 6''$ $\quad L = 10$ ft
$t = \frac{1}{2}''$ $\quad w = 50$ lb/ft
$E = 30 \times 10^6$ psi

1. Which of the following most closely approximates the moment diagram of the beam above?

a.

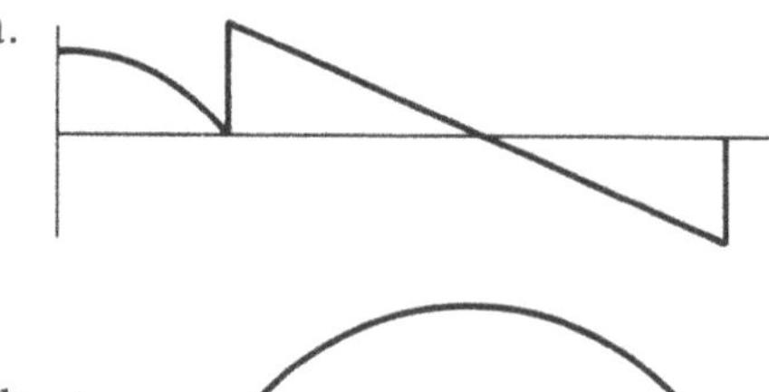

b.

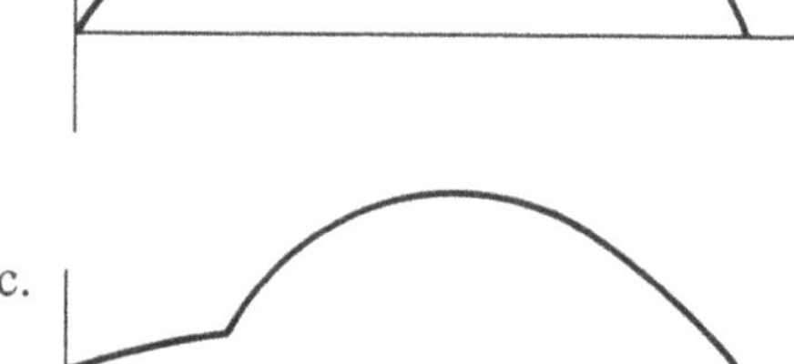

c.

d.

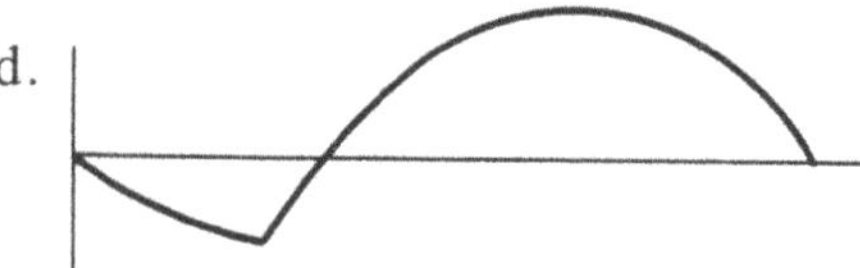

e.

2. $\bar{y} = ?$

   a. 2.2 in.
   b. 4.3 in.
   c. 3.8 in.
   d. 2.7 in.
   e. 5.6 in.

3. $I_{xx} = ?$

   a. 19.9 $in.^4$.
   b. 28.3 $in.^4$.
   c. 22.3 $in.^4$.
   d. 17.6 $in.^4$.
   e. 15.1 $in.^4$.

4. $I_{yy} = ?$

   a. 9.0 $in.^4$.
   b. 4.5 $in.^4$.
   c. 5.3 $in.^4$.
   d. 8.0 $in.^4$.
   e. 1.5 $in.^4$.

5. How far from the left end will the moment be maximum?

   a. 7.2 ft.
   b. 5.8 ft.
   c. 6.2 ft.
   d. 8.9 ft.
   e. 10.3 ft.

6. M_{max} is closest to:

   a. 300 lb-ft.
   b. 500 lb-ft.
   c. 700 lb-ft.
   d. 900 lb-ft.
   e. 1100 lb-ft.

7. The formula for maximum shearing stress is:

   a. $S = Mc/I$.
   b. $S = Tc/j$.
   c. $S = VQ/It$.
   d. $S = EE$.
   e. $S = \pi^2 EI/e^2$.

8. Maximum tensile stress is closest to:

   a. 304 psi.
   b. 684 psi.
   c. 2350 psi.
   d. 128 psi.
   e. 3500 psi.

9. Remove that part of the beam to the left of the left support, making it a simply supported, uniformly loaded beam. The deflection at mid-span is:

   a. 69.1×10^{-6} in.
   b. 49.3×10^{-4} in.
   c. 76.7×10^{-8} in.
   d. 83.1×10^{-9} in.
   e. 64.4×10^{-7} in.

10. The maximum moment for the beam described in question 9 is:

    a. 7500 lb-in.
    b. 6400 lb-in.
    c. 3600 lb-in.
    d. 1800 lb-in.
    e. 9800 lb-in.

Check your answers.

Answers

1. b.
2. b.
3. a.
4. a.
5. d.
6. d.
7. c.
8. c.
9. c.
10. a.

17 Electricity

Discussion of and problems related to electrical work, resistance, batteries, resistance networks, magnetism, electromagnetic induction, capacitance, alternating current, Ohm's Law applied to ac circuits, complex notation, three-phase power, and resonant circuits.

A. INTRODUCTION

Electrical phenomena are based on the charge of an electron. When one or more of the valence electrons are removed from an atom, a positive ion is formed. This ion tends to attract electrons. Conversely, an excess of valence electrons results in a negative ion which tends to give up electrons. These ions are said to have electric charges. The unit of charge (Q) is the coulomb:

$$1\ \text{C} = 6.28 \times 10^{18}\ \text{electrons.}$$

The force of attraction or rejection of electrons is based on Coulomb's Law.

Coulomb's Law in the mks system:

$$F = \frac{1}{4\pi E}\,\frac{Q_1 Q_2}{d^2},$$

where
F is in Newtons,
E is the permittivity of the surrounding medium (8.85×10^{-12} for air)
d is the distance between charges in meters

Example

What is the force between two electrons separated by one meter?

$$F = \frac{1}{4\pi E} \frac{Q_1 Q_2}{d_2}$$

$$= \frac{(1.6 \times 10^{-19})^2}{4\pi(8.85 \times 10^{-12})}$$

$$= 2.3 \times 10^{-28} \text{ N.}$$

Since the charges are of like sign, this is a repelling force.

PROBLEM

What is the force created between two bodies separated by 1 ft when each body has a positive charge of 2 coulombs?

a. 87×10^9 lb attraction.
b. 87×10^9 lb repulsion.
c. 387×10^9 lb attraction.
d. 387×10^9 lb repulsion.
e. None of the above.

Check your answer.

Answer

b.

B. ELECTRICAL WORK

A single charge has the potential for causing a force on any other charged particle nearby. A charge in space then is said to have an electric field, a vector:

$$\vec{E} = \vec{F}/Q \text{(Newtons/coulomb = volts/metre).}$$

This leads to the definition of the basic electrical unit, the *volt*. The work done in moving an electric charge in an electrical field is defined by the following relationship:

$$\Delta E = \frac{W}{Q} = \int E \cos \theta \, d\ell,$$

where

E is in volts,
W is in joules or watt-sec, and
$\cos \theta \, d\ell$ is the movement with respect to the vector.

The work can also be expressed in engineering units:

$$W = 0.738 Q \, \Delta E \text{ (ft-lb).}$$

Since force is required to move a charged electron in an electric field with a potential E, it follows that in the absence of force, the electron will be caused to move. Such a flow of electrons is defined as current (I) measured in amperes.

$$I = \frac{dQ}{dt} \left(\frac{\text{coulombs}}{\text{sec}} = \text{amps} \right).$$

The rate of charge of work with respect to time is power.

> Electrical Power:
>
> Volts and amps are related to the concept of power when both current and potential are steady:
>
> $$P = \frac{dW}{dt} = \frac{d(Q,E)}{dt} = E\frac{dQ}{dt} = EI.$$
>
> If potential E is in volts and current I is in amps, power P is in watts.

Example

A 120-V dc motor is used to lift 1000 lb 44.25 ft in 1 min. How much current is required?

$$I = \frac{P}{E} = \frac{(1000)(44.25)\text{ ft-lb}}{(60)\text{ sec }(120)\text{ V}} \times 1.356 \frac{\text{J}}{\text{ft-lb}}$$

$$= 8.33 \frac{\text{J}}{\text{sec-V}} = 8.33 \frac{\text{W}}{\text{V}} = 8.33 \text{ A}.$$

PROBLEMS

1. Which of the following is *not* a legitimate unit of power?

   a. J/sec.
   b. Ft-lb/sec.
   c. W-h.
   d. Erg/sec.
   e. V-A.

2. The electric field one meter from an electron is:

   a. 2.3×10^{-28} N.
   b. 23×10^{-32} N.
   c. 1.62×10^{-8} dyne/C.
   d. 14.4×10^{-10} N/C.
   e. 1.44×10^{-12} N/C.

Check your answers.

Answers

1. c.
2. d.

C. RESISTANCE

All metals are of a crystalline structure. Chemically the bond between atoms or molecules is covalent. In a covalent bond the electrons are shared, i.e., relatively free to move around within the solid. Hence, if extra electrons are added to one end of a metal, the same number can be removed from the other end. This is *electric current.*

The relative ease of moving electrons through a conductor depends on:

- cross-sectional area;
- length;
- freedom of electrons to move (a function of the metal).

The last factor, the freedom of electrons to move, is called *resistivity*, which is a function of the material.

Total resistance is a combination of these three factors. It is also the ratio of the volts per unit current flow.

Ohm's Law:

$$R = E/I \ (\Omega\text{-ohms})$$

Example

40 V cause a 2-A current to flow through a conductor. Resistance is

$$R = \frac{40}{2} = 20 \ \Omega.$$

What is the change in resistance if the cross-sectional area is doubled?

Resistivity is

$$\rho = R\frac{A}{\ell} = \text{constant.}$$

Therefore,

$$\frac{R_1}{R_2} = \frac{A_2}{A_1}.$$

Resistance is reduced by half.

PROBLEMS

1. Which of the following is a legitimate unit of resistivity?

   a. In.$^3/\Omega$.
   b. Ω/circular mil-ft

c. Ω/mil^3.
d. Ω-ft/circular mil.
e. Ω/ft.

2. The net resistance of the following network is nearest to:

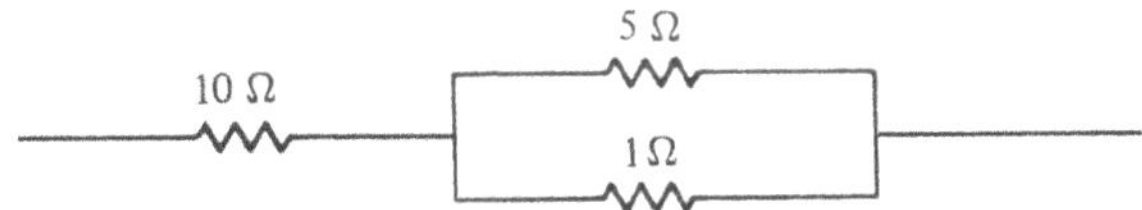

a. 16 Ω.
b. 14 Ω.
c. 11 Ω.
d. 9 Ω.
e. 13 Ω.

Check your answers.

Answers

1. b.
2. c.

D. BATTERIES

Consider the common lead-acid battery consisting of a vessel of sulphuric acid and two electrodes, one lead and one lead peroxide:

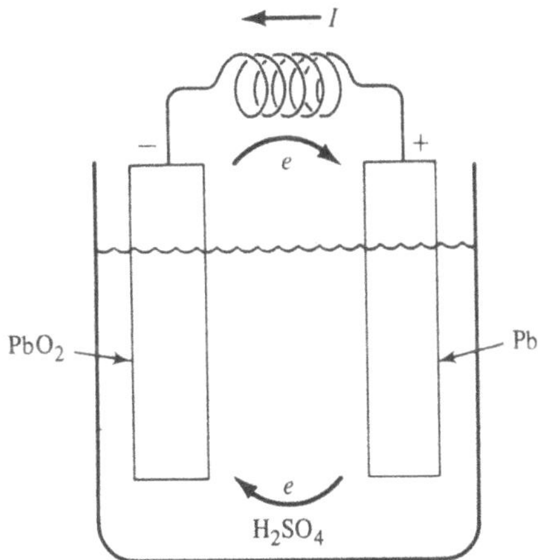

Note that the conventional current flow is opposite the flow of electrons. When a circuit is completed external to the battery, electrons will flow. These are the valence electrons which change partners in a chemical reaction. The reaction is

$$PbO_2 + Pb + 2H_2SO_4 \longrightarrow 2PbSO_4 + 2H_2O.$$

As the battery is discharged, the electrodes are coated with lead sulfate, and the acid becomes weaker.

Each lead-acid cell has a potential of approximately 2 V, depending on the level of charge. Several cells in series will yield a higher voltage.

Graphically:

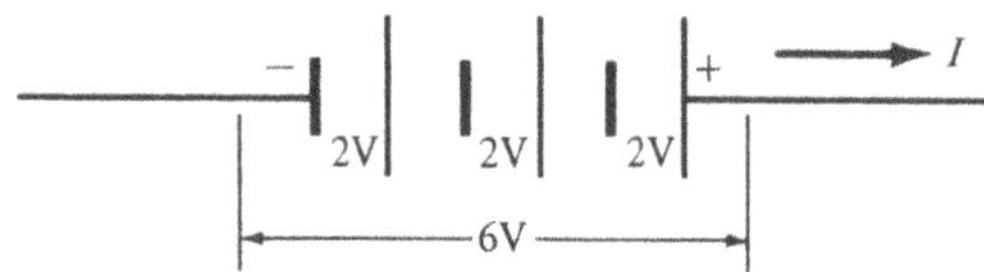

Since the flow of electrons within a battery is not completely free, the battery is said to have internal resistance.

> A *battery* is a chemical producer of emf characterized by two parameters: (1) its open-circuit voltage and (2) its internal resistance.

Example

A battery with an open circuit voltage of 1.5 V and an internal resistance of 0.003 Ω will produce the following emf when delivering 30 A:

$$V = E - IR = 1.5 - (30)(0.003) = 1.5 - .09 = 1.41 \text{ V}.$$

PROBLEMS

1. The energy stored in a battery can be expressed in:

   a. W.
   b. $C^2 - \Omega/\text{sec}$.
   c. J/sec.
   d. Erg/hr.
   e. N/m^2.

2. The current in the circuit shown below is:

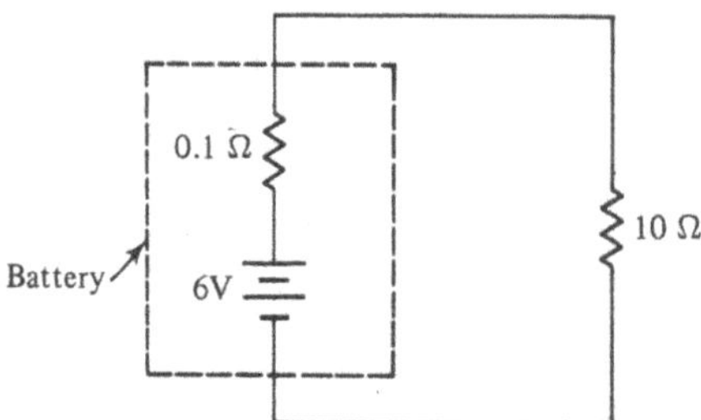

a. 0.606 clockwise.
b. 0.606 counterclockwise.
c. 0.594 clockwise.
d. 0.594 counterclockwise.
e. None of the above.

Check your answers.

Answers

1. b.
2. c.

E. RESISTANCE NETWORKS

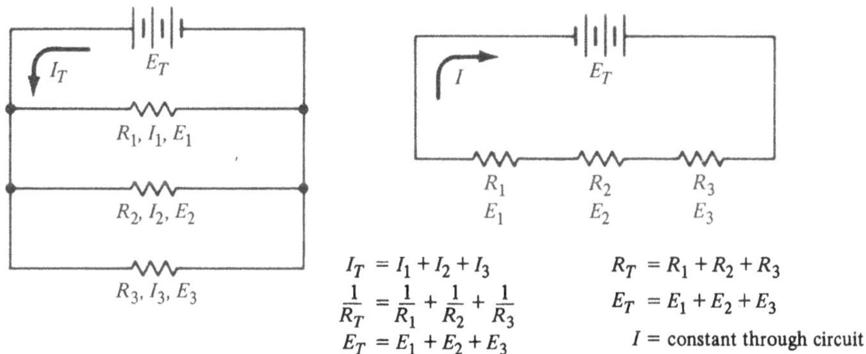

Kirchhoff's Laws

The sum of the currents flowing *toward* a junction point of a circuit equals the sum of the currents flowing *away from* that point. If a plus (+) sign is assigned to currents flowing away from it, then the law states that the algebraic sum of the currents at a junction point is zero:

$$\Sigma I = 0 \quad \text{(at junction point).}$$

In essence, the law simply says that electric charge cannot accumulate at a point, i.e., as much current must flow away as flows toward a point.

The sum of the emfs (rises of potential) around any closed loop of a circuit equals the sum of the potential drops in that loop. Considering a rise of potential as positive (+) and a drop of potential as negative (-), the algebraic sum of the potential differences (voltages) around a closed loop of a circuit is zero:

$$\Sigma E - \Sigma IR \text{ drops} = 0 \quad \text{(around closed loop).}$$

To apply this law, assume an arbitrary current direction for each branch current. The end of the resistor through which the current enters is then positive with respect to the other end. If the solution for the current being solved is negative, then the direction of that current is opposite to the direction assumed.

Kirchhoff's Laws:

1. The sum of the currents at a junction equals 0.
2. The sum of all voltage changes in a loop equals 0.

Example

Find the current through resistor R_1 and the voltage drop across R_1 in the circuit below.

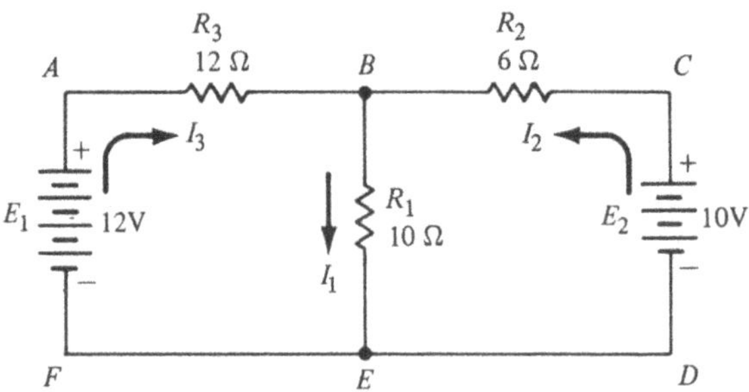

By Kirchhoff's first law, at point B,

$$I_2 + I_3 = I_1 \quad \text{or} \quad I_1 - I_2 - I_3 = 0. \tag{1}$$

By Kirchhoff's second law, the sum of the voltages around loop $EBAFE$ is

$$I_1R_1 + I_3R_3 - E_1 = 0 \quad \text{or} \quad 10I_1 + 12I_3 - 12\text{ V} = 0. \tag{2}$$

The sum of the voltages around loop $EBCDE$ is

$$I_1R_1 + I_2R_2 - E_2 = 0 \quad \text{or} \quad 10I_1 + 6I_2 - 10\text{ V} = 0. \tag{3}$$

We now have three simultaneous equations in three unknowns (I_1, I_2, and I_3). Solving Eq. (1) for I_3 and substituting in Eq. (2),

$$I_3 = I_1 - I_2,$$

and (2) becomes

$$10I_1 + 12(I_1 - I_2) - 12\text{ V} = 0.$$

Simplifying:

$$22I_1 - 12I_2 - 12\text{ V} = 0.$$

Divided by 2:

$$11I_1 - 6I_2 - 6\text{ V} = 0.$$

PROBLEMS

1. The value of the unknown resistance in the wheatstone bridge shown on the next page when the bridge is nulled is:

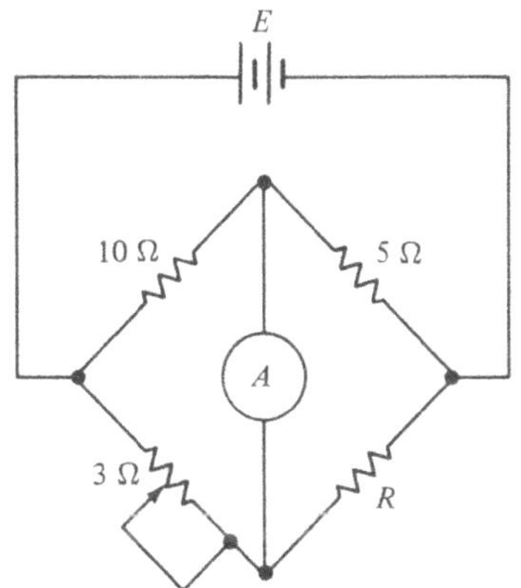

a. 0.66 Ω. c. 6 Ω. e. 1.5 Ω.
b. 1.25 Ω. d. 7.5 Ω.

2. In the circuit below, the current through the 3-Ω resistor is:

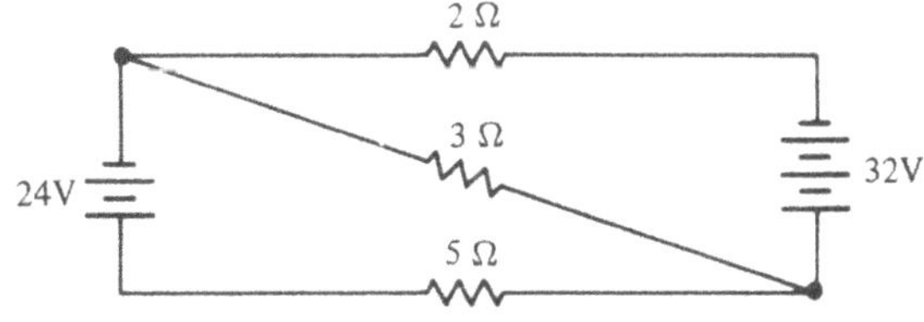

a. 6.8 A. c. 7.2 A. e. 10.6 A.
b. 5.1 A. d. 3.6 A.

Check your answers.

Answers

1. e.
2. c.

F. MAGNETISM

The atomic model assumes that each electron orbits its nucleus and also spins on its axis. In a complete electron shell, half of the electrons spin clockwise; half spin counterclockwise. However, in an incomplete outer shell, more electrons can spin one way than another. For example, in the highly magnetic material, iron, atomic number 26:

1st shell—2 electrons—1cc 1ccw;
2nd shell—8 electrons—4cc 4ccw;
3rd shell—14 electrons—9cc 5ccw;
4th shell—2 electrons—1cc 1ccw.

Each spinning electron produces a spinning electric field which is a vector quantity. Therefore, the vector result of a spinning electron is an electric field vector directed along the spin axis.

In the third shell, where these vectors are not all balanced by oppositely directed spin vectors, the net result is an orbiting, tangentially directed vector. The orbiting vector produces a field vector perpendicular to the plane of orbit; thus each atom with an incomplete shell of electrons produces an electric field vector. Accordingly, two atoms brought together will tend to attract or repel each other depending on the alignment of the vectors. This is the magnetic effect.

In an ordinary iron crystal, the atoms are oriented at random, so the effects of each atomic magnet tend to cancel out. But if the atoms are all aligned either mechanically or with a magnetic field, then each atom's magnetic field reinforces the others, and a permanent magnet with two magnetic poles results.

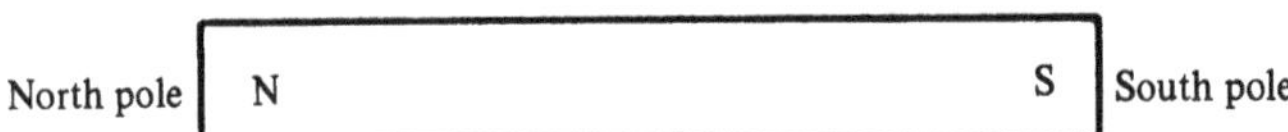

When a current is passed through a coil of wire, exactly the same vector relationships produce a magnetic field with direction perpendicular to the plane of the coil.

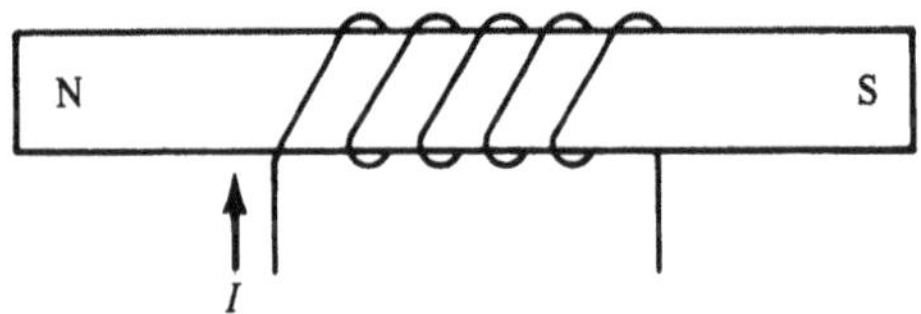

In any magnet, be it a natural magnet or an electromagnet, the forces involved are defined by a magnetic field (a vector quantity analagous to the electric field). Suppose we slowly move a charge Q into the proximity of an uncharged magnet. No electrostatic forces exist. Now suppose we move the particle with charge Q through the field with velocity (v). We now notice a force on the particle. The magnetic field is described by the flux density (B) and is related by the following equation:

$$F = QvB.$$

In the cgs system	*In the SI system*
B is in Gauss	B is in Webers/meter^2
v is in centimetres/second	v is in meters/second
F is in dynes	F is in Newtons

Since F, v, and B are all vectors, the above is a cross-product relationship with vector directions described by the right-hand rule.

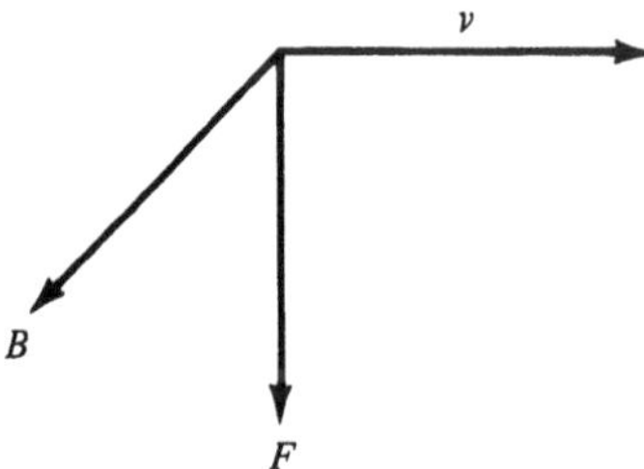

NOTE: Orthogonal axes. When vectors are not orthogonal, the relationship is:

$$F = Q \sin\theta\, B,$$

where θ is the angle between v and B.

Within the permanent magnet or within the core of the electromagnet, the vector B is along the axis. However, in the surrounding air, the direction of the flux density can be envisioned by flux lines emanating from the poles of the magnet. This is known as a magnetic field, symbolized by H (oersteds).

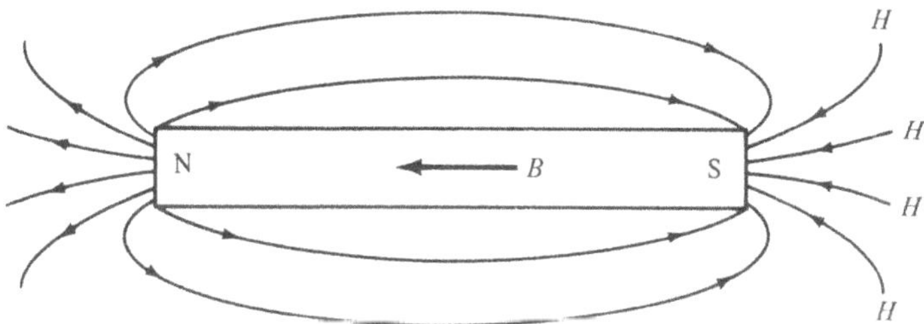

If a magnetic core is inserted into a solenoid, magnetic lines of force will follow the core. The density of these lines of force is called magnetic flux (B) measured in Gauss in the cgs system:

$$B = \mu H,$$

where

μ = permeability of the magnetic core;

H = field intensity in oersteds.

If a current-carrying conductor is located in a magnetic field, it will experience a force in the direction shown:

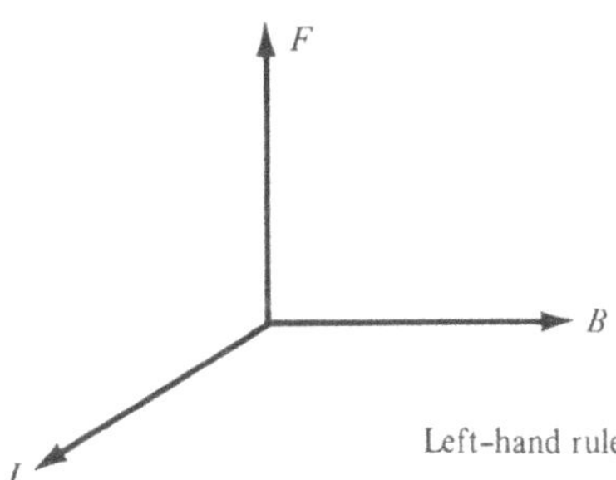

Magnetism:

Force on a charged particle due to a magnetic flux:

$$F = QvB,$$

where v is the velocity on the particle.

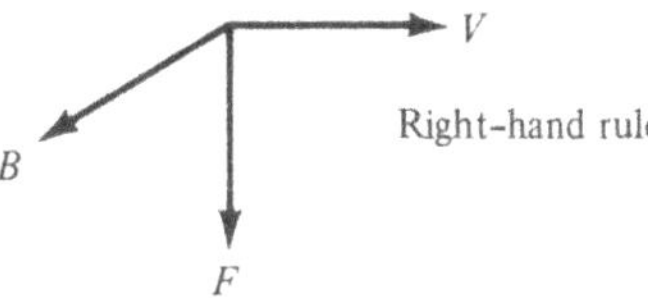

Force on a current-carrying wire:

$$F = IlB,$$

where l is the distance between the magnet and the wire.

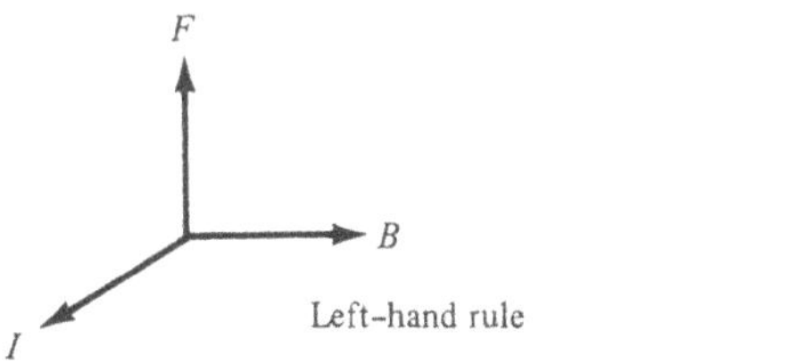

Example

A magnetic field is produced by a coil of wire. An electric current, i.e., charges in motion, is always surrounded by a magnetic field. Consider an elementary (infinitesimal) length dl of a wire carrying a current I. The contribution of the element dl to the magnetic field dH at a point P at a distance r from the wire element is

$$dH = \frac{I \sin \theta \, dl}{r^2},$$

where

I is in amperes;
H is in oersteds;
l is in centimeters;
r is in centimeters; and
θ is the angle between the line r joining the wire element dl to point P and the direction of the current (the tangent at dl). To obtain the total field intensity H at point P, the elementary contributions to the field must be summed up along the entire length of the wire; that is, the expression for dH above must be integrated:

$$H = \int \frac{I \sin \theta}{r^2} \, dl.$$

The expression can be evaluated for various wire configurations such as a single coil on a circular loop.

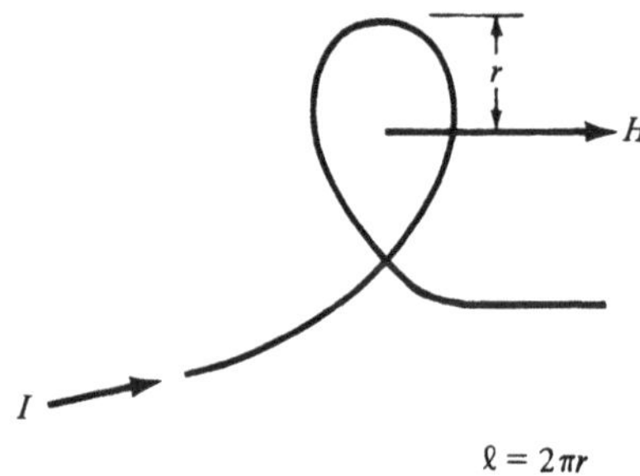

Therefore, integration yields

$$H = \frac{2\pi I}{r} \text{ oersteds.}$$

This is the basis for a torus or a solinoid.

PROBLEMS

1. Which of the following statements is *not* correct?

   a. The north poles of two permanent magnets will repel each other.
   b. A wire with a dc current flowing through it will be surrounded by a magnetic field directed parallel to the wire.
   c. A charged particle traveling perpendicular to the axis near the north pole of a magnet will be deflected in a direction perpendicular to the magnet's axis.

d. The direction of torque in the wheel shown below is clockwise.

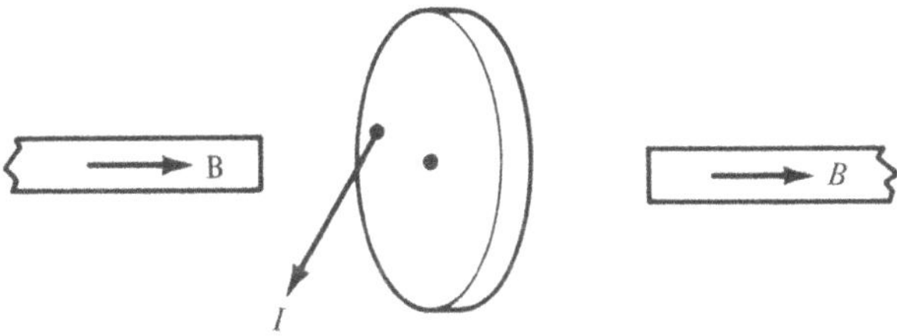

e. Magnetic fields can only be considered vectors very near the pole of an electromagnet.

2. Which of the following expressions is the correct formula for the magnetic field in a long solenoid?

a. $H = 2\pi I/10r$.
b. $H = F/Il\mu$.
c. $H = F/Qv\mu$.
d. $H = 4\pi NI/10l$.
e. $H = 2\pi NI/10r$.

Check your answers.

Answers

1. b.
2. e.

G. ELECTROMAGNETIC INDUCTION

Moving a current-carrying wire through a magnetic field creates a force on the wire. This is the principle of an electric motor.

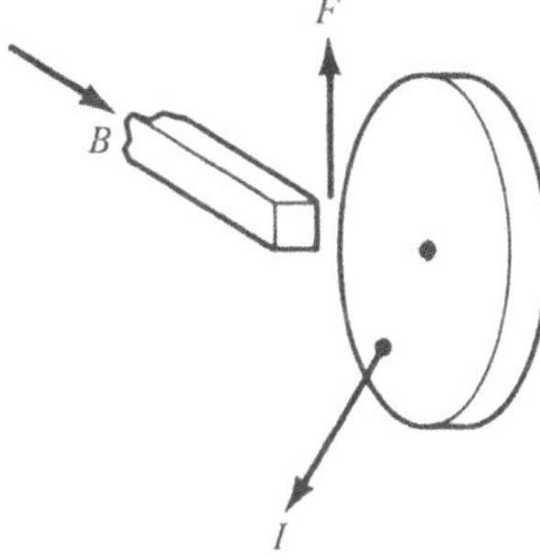

If instead we were to force the armature through the magnetic field, a current would be induced in the wire. This is the principle of a generator. Since the wire is cutting the magnetic lines of force at an angle that varies sinusoidally, the current varies sinusoidally. Hence, this generator produces alternating current.

In the generator the magnetic flux perceived by the wire varies as a function of time. This is a requirement for induced currents. A magnetic field can be varied by other than mechanical means, however. For example, consider two parallel wires. A non-steady-state current in one will induce a non-steady-state current in the other because the magnetic field is also not steady-state.

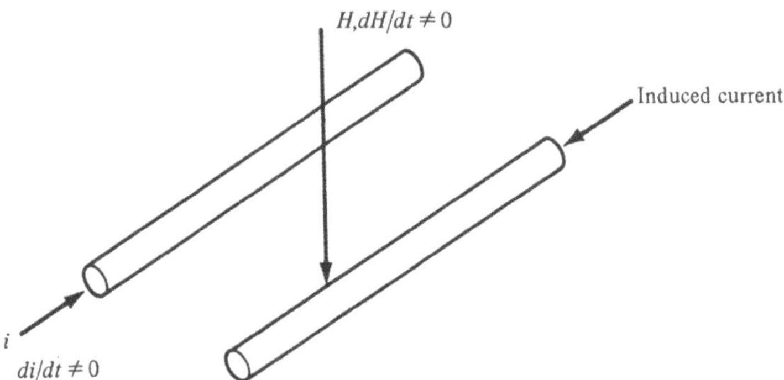

A current passing through a finite-length coil or solenoid changing with time ($I\ di/dt$) is analogous to a current-carrying conductor moving through a field ($I\ dl/dt$) and a secondary emf is induced in the coil. This induced emf is proportional to the rate of current change:

$$E = -L\frac{di}{dt}, \qquad L = \text{inductance (henries).}$$

The negative sign indicates that the emf opposes the change in current, i.e., a counter emf. The inductance of a multiturn solenoid is

$$L = \frac{4\pi N^2 \mu A}{l} \times 10^{-9} \text{ henries}$$

where

N = number of turns,
A = cross-sectional area of core,
μ = permeability of core,
l = length of solenoid.

Inductance is analogous to resistance in an alternating-current circuit where $di/dt \neq 0$.

If two coils are placed next to each other with a common core, current flowing through one coil will induce an emf in the other. This is known as mutual inductance and is the principle of a transformer.

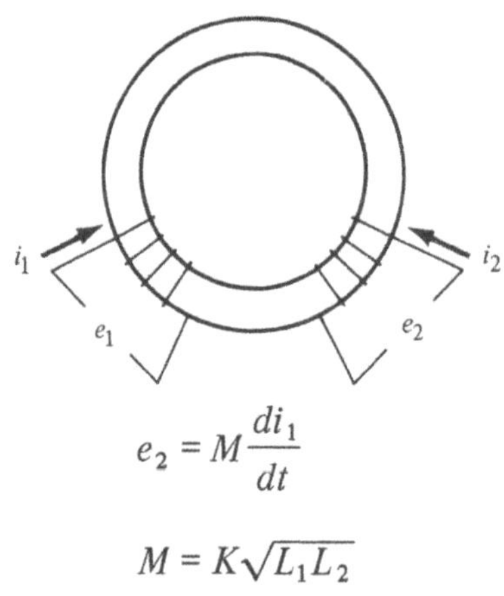

$$e_2 = M\frac{di_1}{dt}$$

$$M = K\sqrt{L_1 L_2}$$

where
M = mutual inductance in henries
K = coefficient of coupling (which approaches unity for a good transformer).

Since inductance of a coil is proportional to the number of turns, in a well-designed transformer

$$\frac{e_1}{e_2} = \frac{N_1}{N_2} \quad \text{and} \quad \frac{i_1}{i_2} = \frac{N_2}{N_1}.$$

Electromagnetic Induction

$$e = -L\frac{di}{dt},$$

where
e is in volts,
L is inductance in henries, and
di/dt is the rate of change of current in Amperes/second.

Example

Consider the RL circuit below:

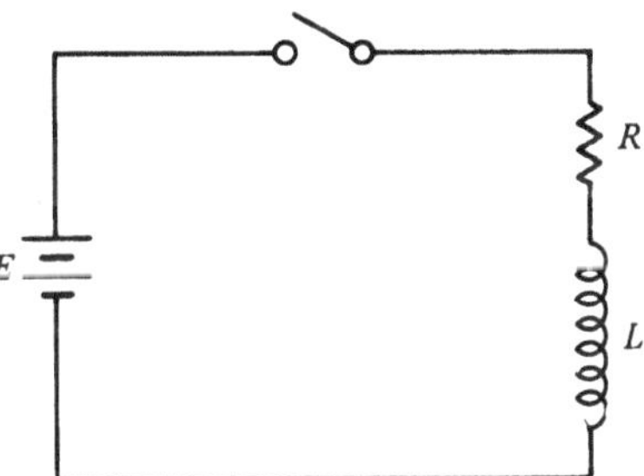

At time 0 the switch is closed. At this time the current is zero. One way to visualize this is that since the electrons have momentum, the current cannot change instantaneously.

At time ∞ the current is steady-state, and the inductor does not impede current flow.

In summary, an inductor acts like an open circuit when current is rapidly changing; it acts like a dead short when current is steady.

Now consider that at some time shortly after the switch is closed:

$$E = Ri + e,$$

or

$$E = Ri - L\frac{di}{dt}$$

where e is the voltage drop across the inductor. Solving the differential equation yields

$$i = E/R(1 - e^{-Rt/L}).$$

Graphically:

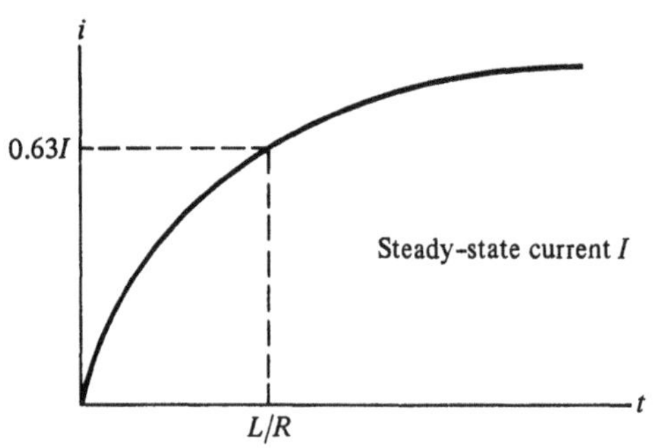

The exponential term L/R, from the above equation called the time constant, is the time required to reach 63% of steady state.

PROBLEMS

1. A transformer has a mutual inductance of 2 henries and a coefficient of coupling of 0.8. The inductances in henries of the two coils are:

   a. 0.37 and 16.25.
   b. 0.25 and 25.
   c. 0.08 and 8.
   d. 0.64 and 128.
   e. 0.727 and 1728.

2. The current in the circuit below 2 seconds after switch closure is closest to:

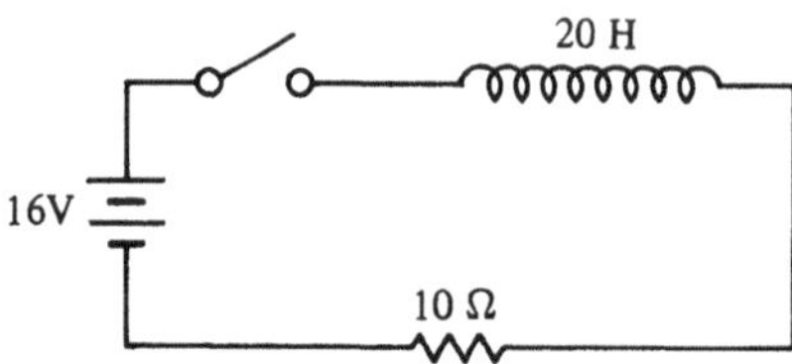

   a. 0.5 A.
   b. 0.75 A.
   c. 1.00 A.
   d. 1.25 A.
   e. 1.50 A.

Check your answers.

Answers

1. b.
2. c.

H. CAPACITANCE

If two conducting surfaces are separated by an insulating material, it is possible to accumulate a charge difference between the two surfaces. Even though an electric field exists, the electrons are prevented from moving by the high resistance of the insulator. Such a device stores electric energy until a circuit of lower resistance is completed between the two surfaces, at which time the electrons flow from one surface to the other through the external circuit producing a current. This describes a capacitor, defined as follows:

$$C = Q/E,$$

where
C = capacitance in farads,
Q = accumulated charge in coulombs,
E = potential between the two surfaces.

When electrostatic charge is added to the two parallel plates, the plates accept a charge until the electrostatic potential is equal to the applied voltage supplying the charge.

When the capacitor is fully charged, its stored energy is

$$W(\text{joules}) = \tfrac{1}{2}CV^2.$$

Capacitance of capacitors in parallel is

$$C_T = C_1 + C_2 + \cdots.$$

Capacitance of capacitors in series is

$$\frac{1}{C_T} = \frac{1}{C_1} + \frac{1}{C_2} + \cdots.$$

Capacitive Time Constant

Consider the following circuit:

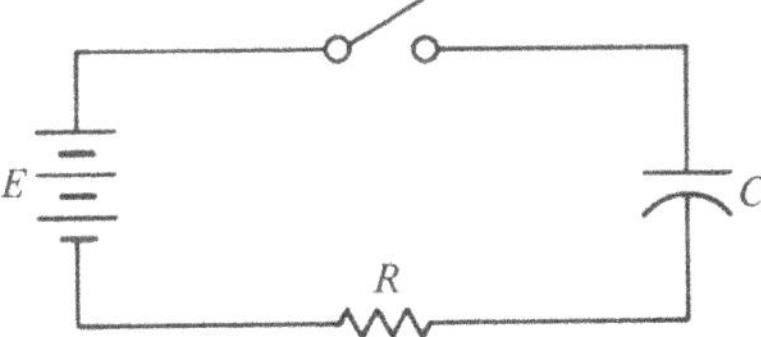

The time required for charging the capacitor to 63.2% of E is:

$$T = RC \text{ (seconds)}.$$

RC is the time constant of the RC circuit.

The time required for 86.5% of E_2 is

$$T = 2RC.$$

This is a way of stating that de/dt represents an exponential curve.

T = 63.2% of charge or discharge
$2T$ = 86.5% of charge or discharge
$3T$ = 95% of charge or discharge
$5T$ = 99.3% of charge or discharge.

Capacitance:

$$C = Q/E$$

where
C = capacitance in farads,
Q = charge in coulombs,
E = potential in volts.

Example

Determine the expression for current in a capacitive circuit as a function of time. Consider the RC circuit below after the switch is closed:

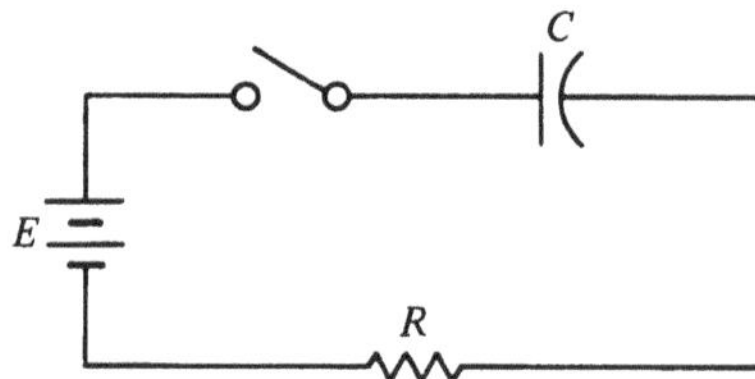

At time 0 the switch is closed. At this time the current is at its maximum value because the capacitor is being charged. At time ∞ the current is zero because the capacitor is fully charged and can absorb no more current. (Note that there is no steady-state continuity through the capacitor.)

In summary, a capacitor acts like a dead short when current is rapidly changing; it acts like an open circuit when the current is steady.

At some time shortly after the switch is closed,

$$V = iR + \frac{Q}{C}$$

or

$$V = iR + \frac{1}{C}\int i\,dt.$$

Solving this differential equation yields

$$i = \frac{V - V_0}{R} e^{-t/RC}.$$

Graphically:

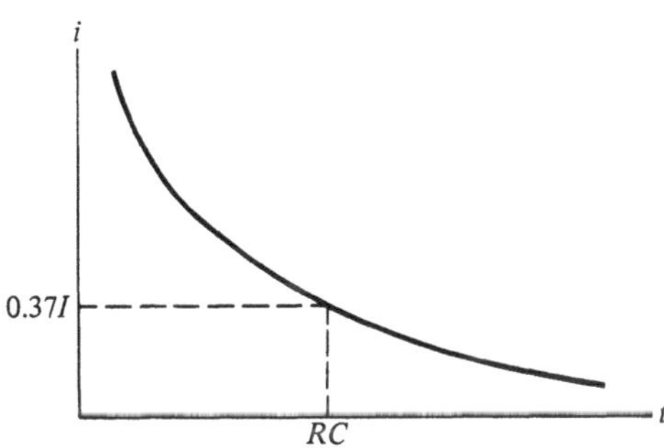

The exponential term RC, called the time constant, is the time required to reach 63% of steady state.

PROBLEMS

1. The capacitor shown below is fully charged when the switch is closed.

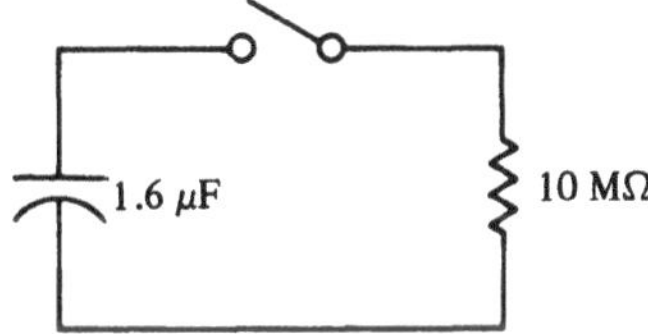

Which of the following curves best describes the time history of the current?

a. i

5 10 15 20 t

b.

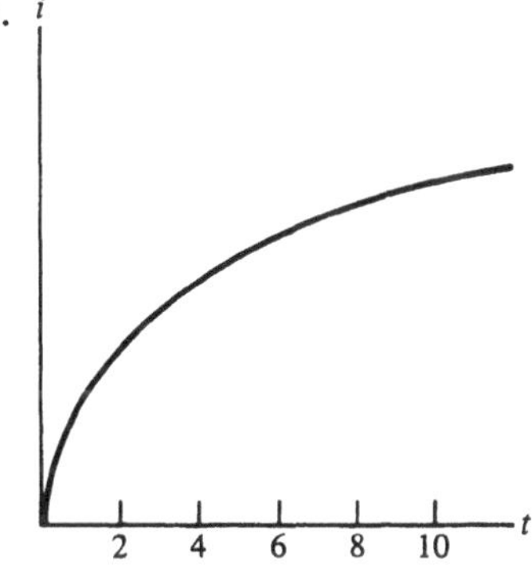

c.

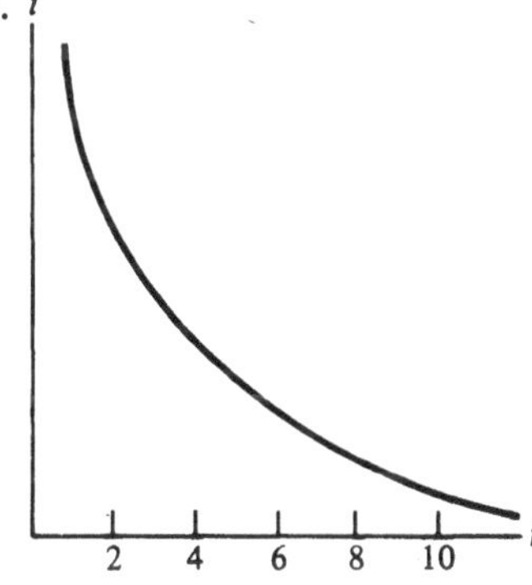

d. i

5 10 15 20 t

e.

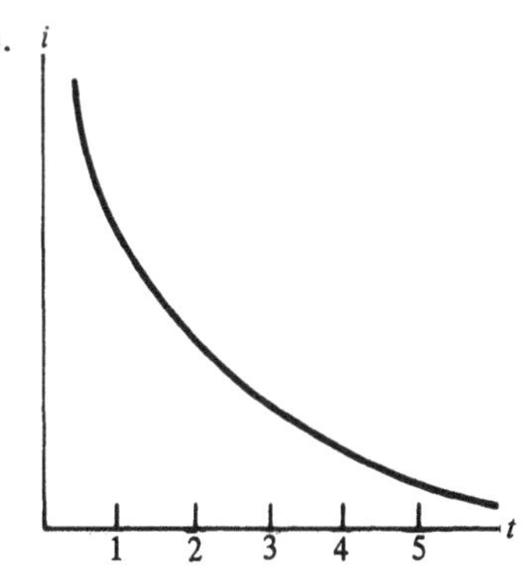

2. In the circuit below, calculate the current drawn from the battery immediately after the switch is closed.

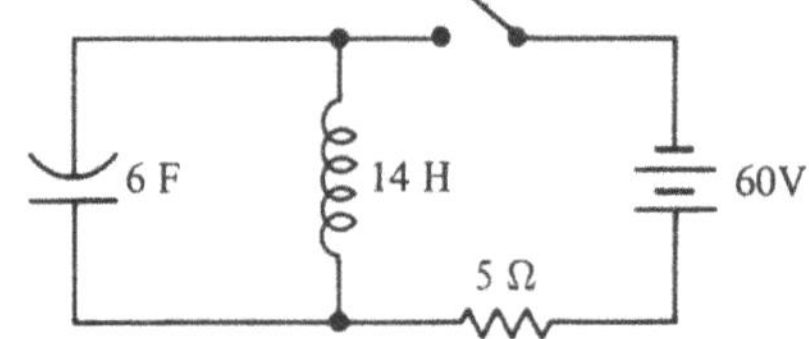

a. 2.4 A. c. 10 A. e. 12 A.
b. 2 A. d. 6 A.

Check your answers.

Answers

1. d.
2. e.

I. ALTERNATING CURRENT

Alternating current is associated with rotating machinery. When a conductor or winding is mounted on a rotating member called an armature, its position with respect to a magnetic field vector varies as

$$y \approx \sin \omega t,$$

where ω is the angular velocity of the armature.

In terms of frequency,

$$\omega = 2\pi f,$$

where f is the frequency in cycles per second or hertz.

Producing an Alternating Current

Consider the following simple alternator with a purely inductive load:

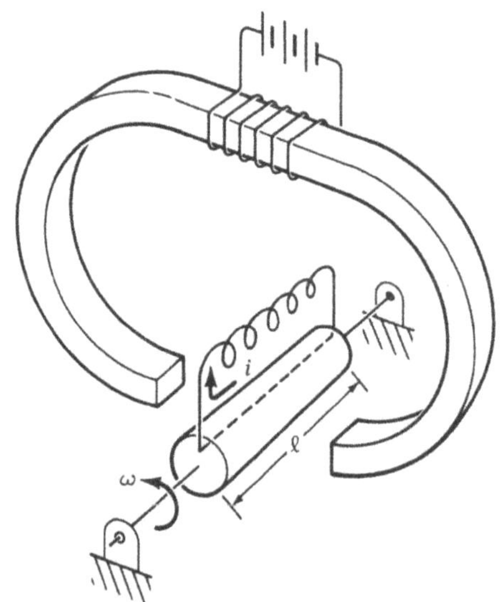

As the armature rotates through the magnetic field with velocity $v = \omega r$, it produces an emf:

$$E = Blv \sin \theta,$$

where θ is on a plane perpendicular to the magnetic lines of force.

E will be maximum positive at $\theta = 0°$.

E will be maximum negative at $\theta = 270°$.

This can be illustrated by the following sketch.

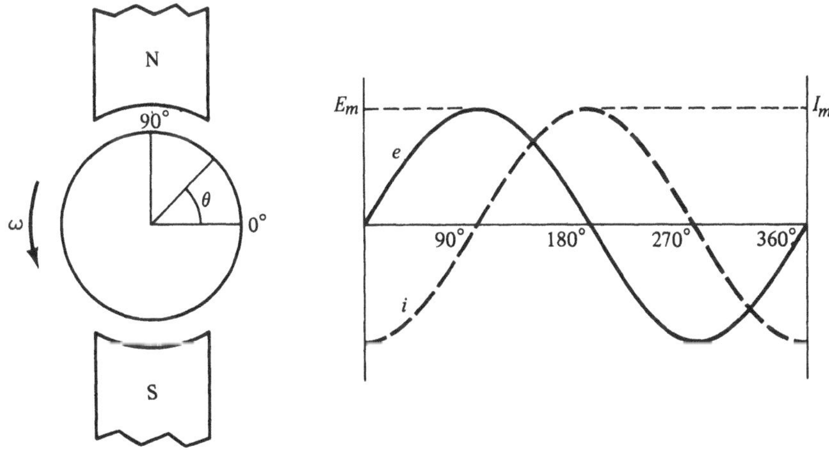

For a given field intensity E is proportional to $v = \omega r$ and phase angle θ:

$$e = E_m \sin \theta = E_m \sin \omega t$$

$$i = I_m \sin (\omega t + \theta).$$

The frequency of the generated current is

$$f = \frac{\omega}{2\pi} \text{ Hz},$$

or for multipoles

$$\text{rpm} = \frac{120f}{\text{No. poles}}.$$

If the above current is passed through a resistor it will produce heat as follows:

$$P = \frac{E_m I_m}{2} = \left(\frac{E_m}{\sqrt{2}}\right)\left(\frac{I_m}{\sqrt{2}}\right)$$

$$\frac{E_m}{\sqrt{2}} = 0.707\, E_m = E_{\text{rms}}.$$

Similarly

$$\frac{I_m}{\sqrt{2}} = 0.707\, I_m = I_{\text{rms}}.$$

In the generator illustrated below, current lags the voltage by 90° because the self inductance in the armature coil opposes the change in current. For the common circuit elements:

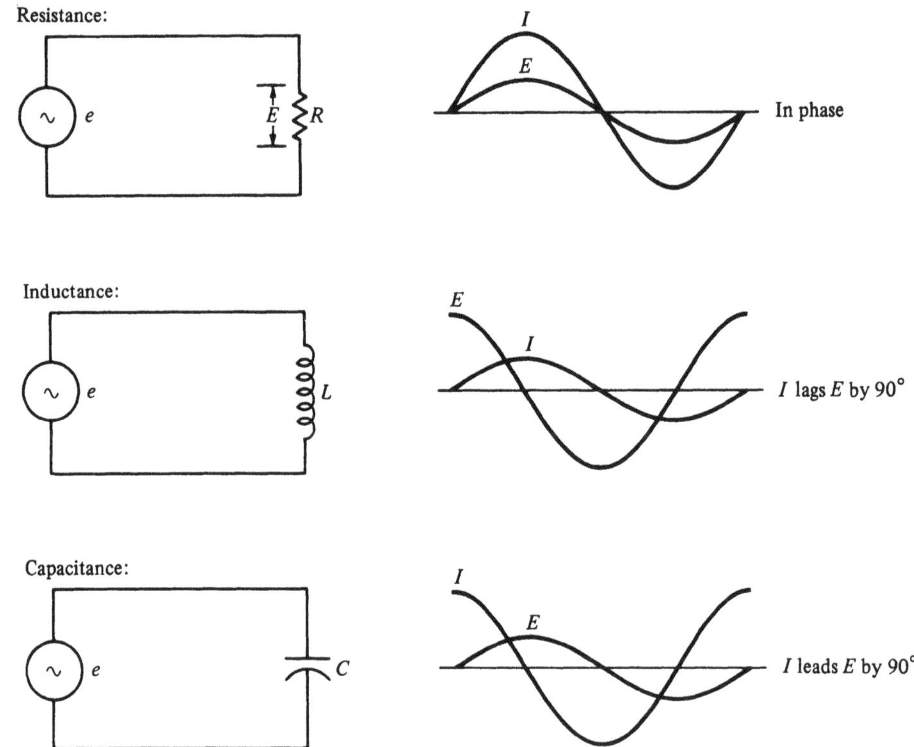

Alternating Current Motors

The mechanism of a motor is exactly the same as an alternator except that, instead of a torque being applied to the armature to produce a current in a motor, a current is impressed to the armature and a torque is produced.

For a two-pole motor, the synchronous speed is

$$\omega = 2\pi f$$

or, in terms of rpm,

$$N = \frac{60\omega}{2\pi} = 60f \quad \text{in rpm.}$$

For a motor of four or more poles,

$$N = \frac{120f}{P},$$

where P is number of poles.

Alternating-Current Generators and Motors:

$$e = E_{max} \sin (\omega t + \theta)$$

$$i = I_{max} \sin (\omega t + \phi)$$

$$w = 2\pi f$$

$$E_{rms} = \frac{E_{max}}{\sqrt{2}}$$

$$I_{rms} = \frac{I_{max}}{\sqrt{2}}.$$

For a resistive load–voltage and current are in phase.
For an inductive load–voltage leads current.
For a capacitive load–current leads voltage.
Synchronous speed of a motor:

$$N = 120f/P.$$

Example

A two-pole alternator is being driven at 1800 rpm. The load has a phase angle such that voltage leads by 60°. Determine the voltage, current, and power relationships.

$$\omega = 2\pi f.$$

Therefore

$$f = \frac{1800}{2\pi}\,\frac{2\pi}{60} = 30 \text{ Hz}$$

$$e = E_{max} \sin 188t$$

$$i = I_{max} \sin (188t + 60).$$

Instantaneous power:

$$P_i = ei \qquad \text{at any point in time.}$$

Average power:

$$P = E_{rms} I_{rms}.$$

Graphically:

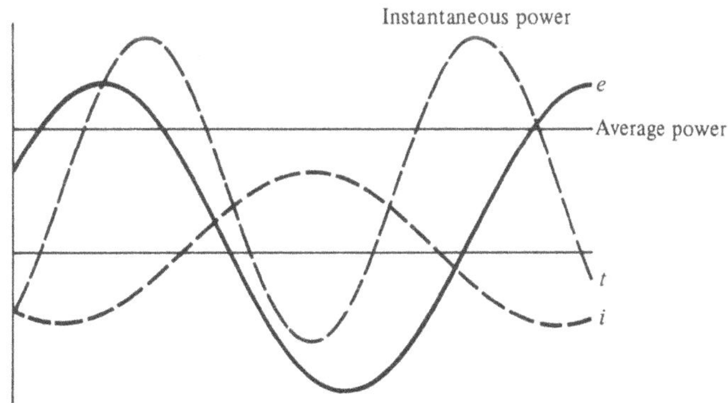

PROBLEMS

1. Given

$$e = 155 \sin 377t$$
$$i = 30 \sin 377t,$$

the heat created by a resistance heater in the circuit is:

a. 4650 W.
b. 2324 W.
c. 1358 W.
d. 2036 W.
e. 1836 W.

2. A single-phase, six-pole motor with 5% slip is operating on 60 Hz current. Its rpm is:

a. 925.
b. 1800.
c. 1725.
d. 1140.
e. 1540.

Check your answers.

Answers

1. b.
2. d.

J. OHM'S LAW APPLIED TO AC CIRCUITS

In addition to resistance, an ac circuit can have two impediments: inductance and capacitance. A term which combines all three impediments to current flow is impedance:

$$Z = \frac{E}{I},$$

where Z is impedance (opposition to current flow). Impedance is the vector sum of the impediments caused by resistance (R), capacitive reactance (X_C), and inductive reactance (X_L).

$$\vec{Z} = \vec{R} + \vec{X}_C + \vec{X}_L.$$

This relationship is expressed as a vector equation because both reactances are 90° opposed to resistance, i.e., they are out of phase. All of the terms in the equation are in ohms (Ω).

The reactive terms are related to frequency and to inductance and capacitance, respectively:

$$X_L = 2\pi f L$$

$$X_C = \frac{1}{2\pi f C}.$$

Since X_C and X_L are 180° opposed, the vector diagram appears as follows:

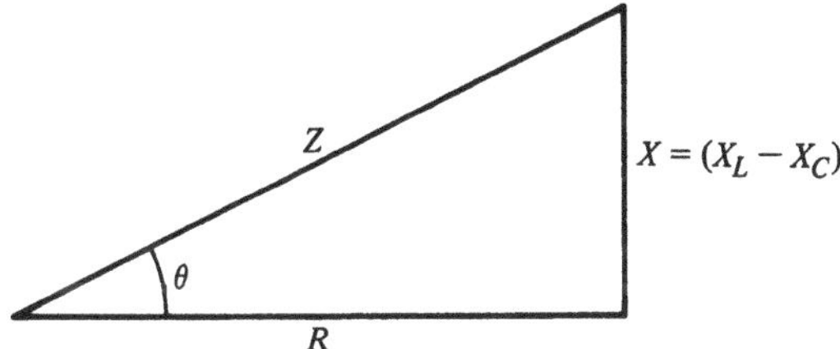

where θ is the phase angle between current and voltage. Here

$$Z = \sqrt{R^2 + \left(2\pi fL - \frac{1}{2\pi fC}\right)^2}$$

and the phase angle θ is given by

$$\theta = \tan^{-1} \frac{X_L - X_C}{R} = \tan^{-1} \frac{2\pi fL - (1/2\pi fC)}{R}.$$

Positive values of θ indicate that current lags voltage.

AC Power

No power is absorbed by capacitors or inductors, but the product of EI is affected by the phase angle at any point in time. Therefore:

$$P = EI \cos \theta.$$

(In power applications $\cos \theta$ is called the power factor–abbreviated pf or ϕ.) Graphically:

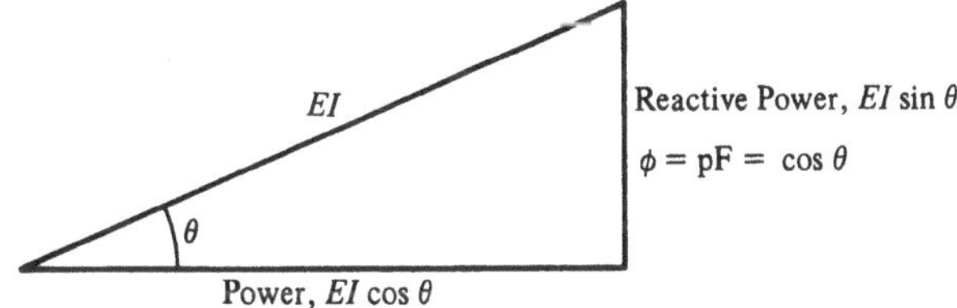

Reactive power does no useful work. Although it is cost-free, as it does not register on the electric meter, it imposes a penalty because transformers and power lines must be sized for the product EI. Therefore, it is desirable to maximize the power factor ($\cos \theta$).

ac Circuits:
Ohm's Law:

$$Z = E/I \; (\Omega).$$

$$\vec{Z} = \vec{R} + (\vec{X}_L - \vec{X}_C)$$

$$\text{Power} = EI \cos \theta$$

$$\text{Power factor} = \cos \theta.$$

Example

What is the power factor of an electric motor operating at 440 V and drawing 8.5 kW at 27.5 A?

$$EI = (440)(27.5) = 12{,}100 \text{ VA}$$

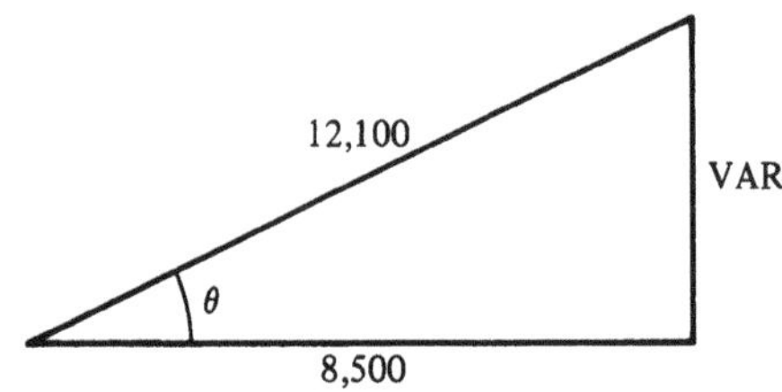

$$\text{VAR} = \sqrt{12{,}100^2 - 8{,}500^2} = 8{,}600$$

$$\phi = \cos\theta = \frac{8{,}500}{12{,}100} = 0.7$$

Suppose it is desired to drop the current to 20 A by adding capacitors and hence increasing the power factor.
New power factor:

$$\phi = \frac{8500}{(440)(20)} = 0.97.$$

What rating capacitor is required?

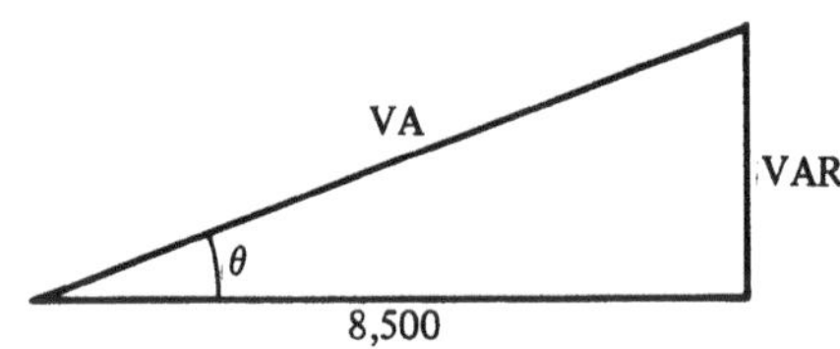

$$\text{VA} = \frac{8500}{0.97} = 8762$$

$$\text{VAR} = \sqrt{8762^2 - 8500^2} = 2130$$

$$\text{Capacitive VAR} = 8600 - 2130 = 6470$$

$$I^2 X_C = 6470.$$

Solve for X_C.

PROBLEMS

1. The impedance of the circuit below is closest to:

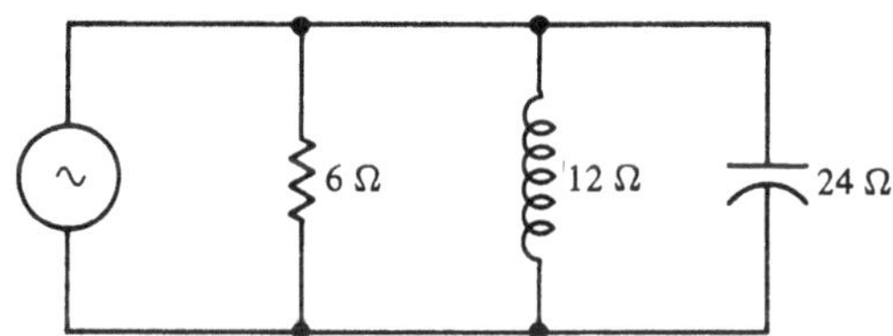

a. 4 Ω.
b. 5 Ω.
c. 6 Ω.
d. 7 Ω.
e. 8 Ω.

2. The total reactance of the following circuit is closest to:

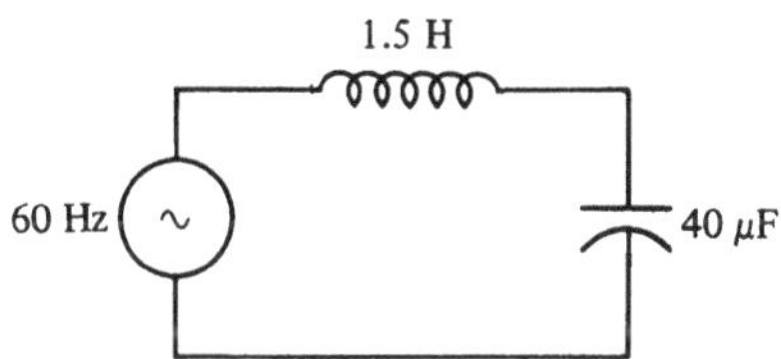

a. 400 Ω inductive.
b. 500 Ω inductive.
c. 600 Ω inductive.
d. 400 Ω capacitive.
e. 500 Ω capacitive.

Check your answers.

Answers

1. c.
2. b.

K. COMPLEX NOTATION

Analysis of a reactive ac circuit is complicated by the necessary consideration of phase angles of different branches. This is most easily done by using complex notation:

Resistance plus inductance: $Z = R + jX_L$

Resistance plus capacitance: $Z = R - jX_C$

The use of the term $j = \sqrt{-1}$ yields a Cartesian relationship in the real and imaginary axes:

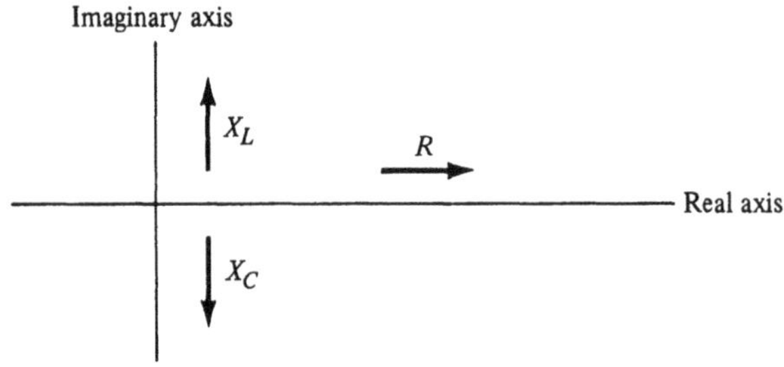

The total impedance can also be written incorporating the inductance and capacitance:

$$Z = R + j\omega L - \frac{j}{\omega C}.$$

Consider the circuit below·

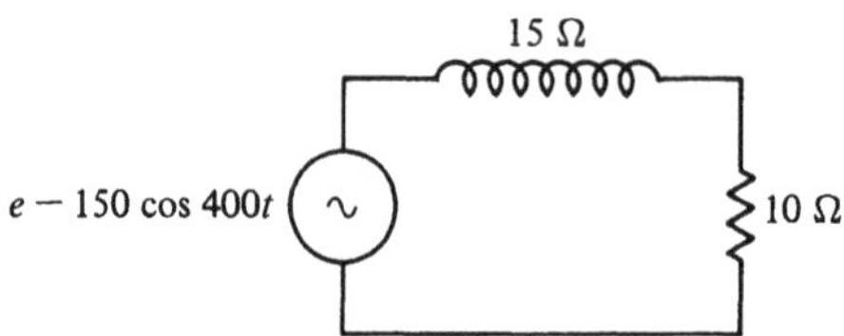

$$\omega = 2\pi f = 400$$

$$X_L = \omega L = 400L = 15\ \Omega.$$

Therefore

$$L = 37.5 \text{ mH}$$

$$e = 150 \cos 400t$$

$$e_{\text{rms}} = \frac{150}{\sqrt{2}} \angle 0^\circ$$

$$= 106 \angle 0^\circ.$$

(The phase angle indicates that 0° is the baseline.)

$$Z = R + jX_L = 10 + j15$$

$$= 18.02 \angle 56.3^\circ$$

because:

$$\sqrt{10^2 + 15^2} = 18.02$$

$$\tan^{-1} \frac{15}{10} = 56.3^\circ.$$

Therefore, the current in this circuit is:

$$i = \frac{e}{Z} = \frac{106\,\angle 0^\circ}{18.02\,\angle 56.3^\circ},$$

which means that $i = 5.9$ A lagging voltage by 56.3°.

Complex Notation:

$$Z = R + jX_L - jX_C$$

or

$$Z = R + j\omega L - \frac{j}{\omega C}.$$

Example

Given the circuit below:

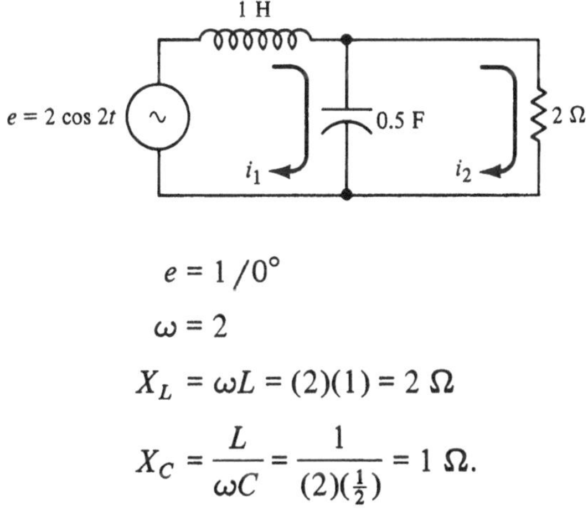

$$e = 1\,\angle 0^\circ$$

$$\omega = 2$$

$$X_L = \omega L = (2)(1) = 2\ \Omega$$

$$X_C = \frac{L}{\omega C} = \frac{1}{(2)(\frac{1}{2})} = 1\ \Omega.$$

Using Kirchhoff's Law, find the current i_1.

In the left loop,

$$1\,\angle 0^\circ = (jX_L - JX_C)i_1 + jX_C i_2.$$

In the right loop,

$$0 = jX_C i_1 + (R - jX_C)i_2.$$

Therefore

$$i_1 = \frac{\begin{vmatrix} 1\,\angle 0^\circ & j \\ 0 & 2-j \end{vmatrix}}{\begin{vmatrix} j & j \\ j & 2-j \end{vmatrix}} = \frac{2-j}{2+j2}.$$

Multiplying by the complex conjugate:

$$i_1 = \frac{2 - j}{2 + j2} \cdot \frac{2 - j2}{2 - j2} = \frac{2 - j6}{8}$$

$$i_1 = 0.790 \underline{/-71.56^\circ} \text{ A}$$

where i_1 lags voltage by 71.56°.

PROBLEMS

1. Another way of stating the current $i = -0.25 - j0.25$ is:

   a. $0.353 \underline{/-135^\circ}$.
   b. $0.706 \underline{/-67.5^\circ}$.
   c. $0.353 \underline{/135^\circ}$.
   d. $0.706 \underline{/-67.5^\circ}$.
   e. None of these.

2. The current in the following circuit is:

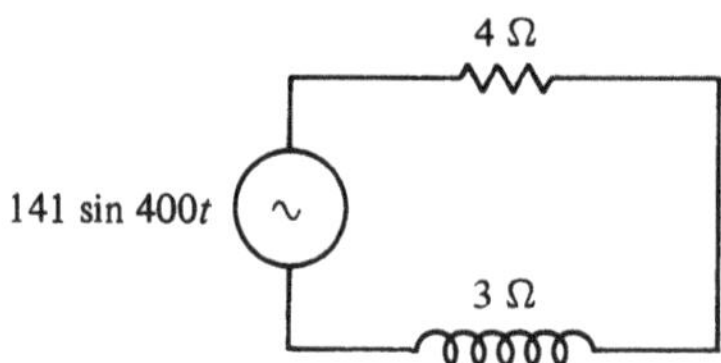

   a. $17 - j23$.
   b. $23 + j17$.
   c. $12 - j16$.
   d. $23 - j17$.
   e. $16 - j12$.

Check your answers.

Answers

1. a.
2. c.

L. THREE-PHASE POWER

Three-phase current results from three separate armature circuits 120° apart. The power-absorbing system can be connected in two ways: the delta (Δ) connection and the wye (Y) connection.

Delta Connection

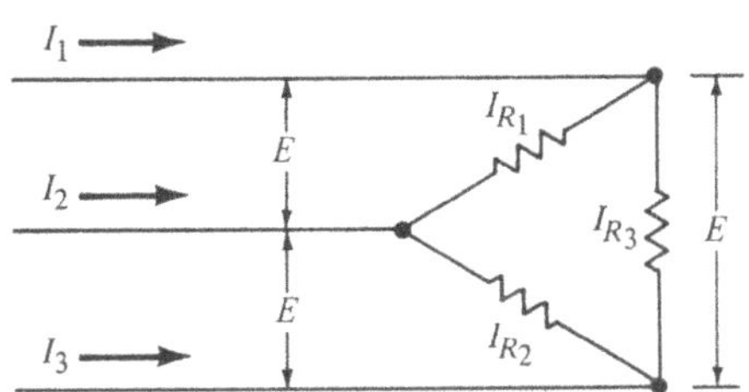

$$I_1 = 2I_{R_1} \sin 120°$$

$$I_1 = I_R\sqrt{3}.$$

Therefore

$$P = 3EI_R$$

$$P = \sqrt{3}\, EI.$$

Y Connection

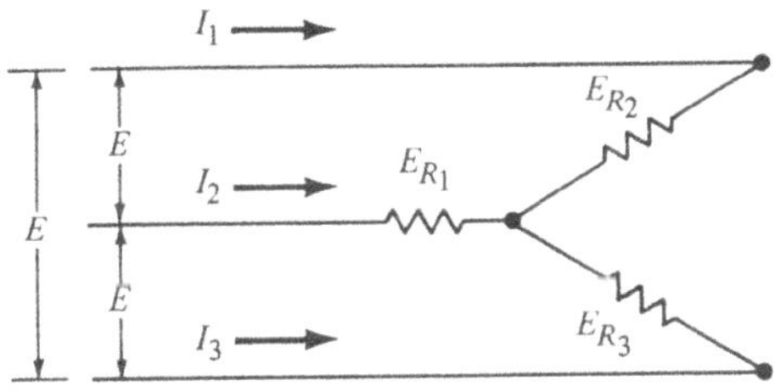

$$E_1 = 2E_{R_1} \sin 120°$$

$$E_1 = E_{R_1}\sqrt{3}.$$

Therefore

$$P = 3IE_R$$

$$P = \sqrt{3}\, EI.$$

> Three-Phase Power:
>
> $$P = \sqrt{3}\, EI$$
>
> for a balanced load, regardless of the connection.

Example

Determine the line current of a 95% efficient 200 hp three-phase motor operating on 440 V ac with a power factor of 0.9.

$$P = \sqrt{3}\, EI \cos\theta$$

$$I = \frac{(200)(746)(1/0.95)}{(\sqrt{3})(440)(0.90)} = 229 \text{ A.}$$

PROBLEMS

1. Given the voltage vector diagram and circuit below, find the phase angle of I_1.

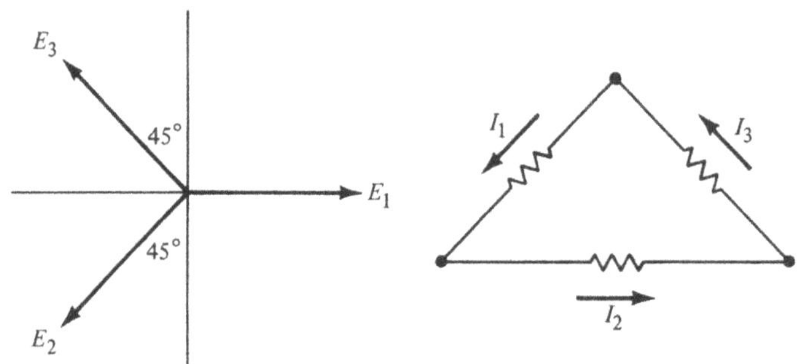

a. -45°.
b. 45°.
c. 195°.
d. 75°.
e. -75°.

2. The impedance of each leg of the equivalent Δ circuit to the circuit shown below is:

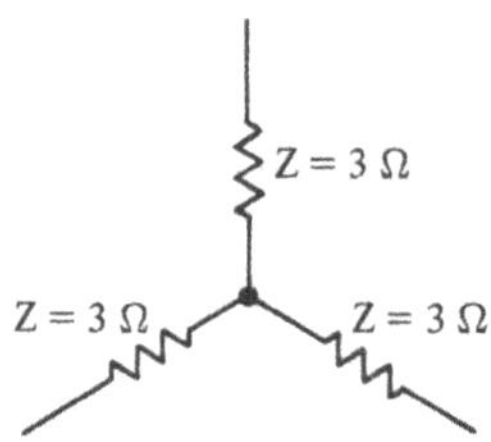

a. 3 Ω.
b. 6 Ω.
c. 9 Ω.
d. 12 Ω.
e. None of the above.

Check your answers.

Answers

1. a.
2. c.

M. RESONANT CIRCUITS

The second-order differential equation describing the LRC circuit is

$$L\frac{d^2q}{dt^2} + \frac{dq}{dt}R + \frac{q}{C} = f(t)$$

where

q is charge in coulombs,
dq/dt is current in amperes,
L is inductance in henries,
R is resistance in ohms, and
C is capacitance in farads.

When the equation is solved for series and parallel combinations of inductance, resistance, and capacitance, we have the equations of a resonant circuit. The material following is based on a solution where $f(t)$ is a sinusoidal source.

Series Resonance

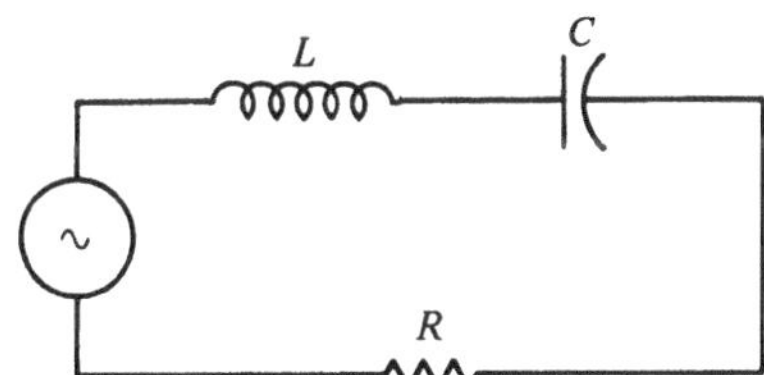

Solving the differential equation for a step input yields the natural frequency of the circuit:

$$\omega_0 = \frac{1}{\sqrt{LC}}.$$

Since $X_C = 1/\omega C$ and $X_L = \omega L$, at this resonant frequency,

$$X_L = X_C.$$

In any RLC circuit, a certain amount of energy is stored in the inductor and in the capacitor. A certain amount of energy is dissipated by the resistor. The ratio of these is called the Figure of Merit.

$$Q = \frac{\text{reactance energy}}{\text{resistance energy}} = \frac{\omega_0 L}{R} = \frac{1}{\omega_0 CR} = \frac{1}{R}\sqrt{\frac{L}{C}}.$$

The Figure of Merit for a circuit can also be defined as the ratio of the natural frequency to the frequency bandwidth which encompasses half of the stored energy:

$$Q = \left.\frac{\omega_0}{\Delta\omega}\right|_{\text{(half power)}}$$

The total current of series circuits as a function of frequency is illustrated as follows:

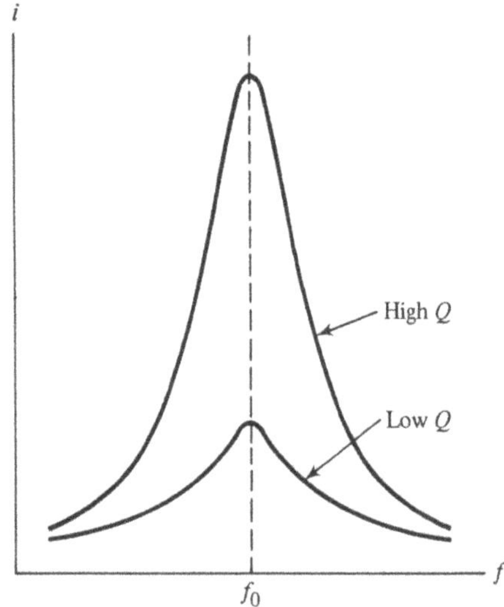

Since $X_L = X_C$ at resonance, the total impedance of the circuit at its natural frequency is $Z = R$.

Parallel Resonance

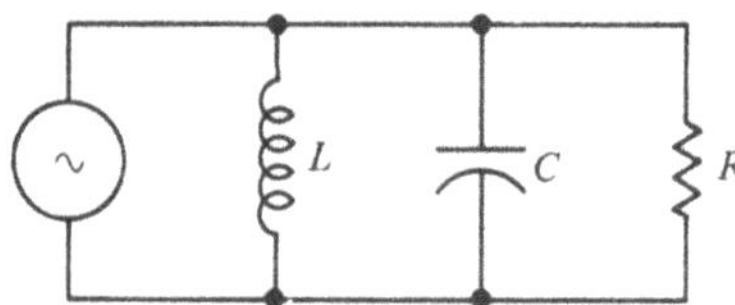

A solution of the differential equation for the above circuit yields the same natural frequency as for a series circuit:

$$\omega_0 = \frac{1}{\sqrt{LC}}.$$

And, as with a series circuit,

$$X_L = X_C.$$

The Figure of Merit is

$$Q = R\sqrt{\frac{C}{L}},$$

which is the ratio of natural frequency to half-power bandwidth, as in the case of series resonance.

In a series resonant circuit, maximum current occurs at the natural frequency; in a parallel circuit, maximum impedance occurs at the natural frequency:

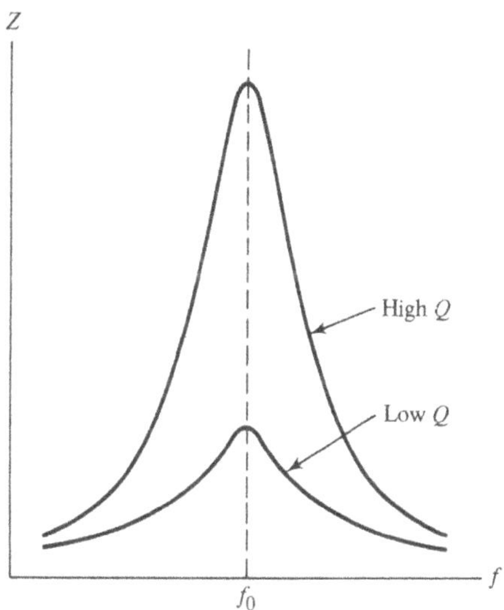

The total impedance of a parallel circuit at resonance is

$$Z = \frac{1}{\frac{1}{R} + j(X_C - X_L)}.$$

Since $X_C = X_L$,

$$Z = R,$$

except in the case where $R = 0$. Then $Z \longrightarrow \infty$.

Series Resonance	*Parallel Resonance*
$\omega_0 = \frac{1}{\sqrt{LC}}$	$\omega_0 = \frac{1}{\sqrt{LC}}$
$X_L = X_C$	$X_L = X_C$
$Q = \frac{1}{R}\sqrt{L/C}$	$Q = R\sqrt{\frac{C}{L}}$

Example

Determine the resistance required in a series resonant circuit with a given natural frequency to produce a given bandwidth between half-power points.

I R L C

$$f_0 = \frac{1}{2\pi\sqrt{LC}}.$$

At f_0,

$$R = Z$$
$$X_L = X_C$$
$$\theta = 0,$$

where $\cos\theta$ is the power factor.

The power is:

at the natural frequency, $P = EI_0$.

at any other frequency, $P = EI'\cos\theta$,

where $\theta = 2\pi(f' - f_0)$.

But, since impedance increases at other frequencies,

$$Z = \sqrt{R^2 + (X_L - X_C)^2},$$

I drops off with a change of frequency, as shown below.

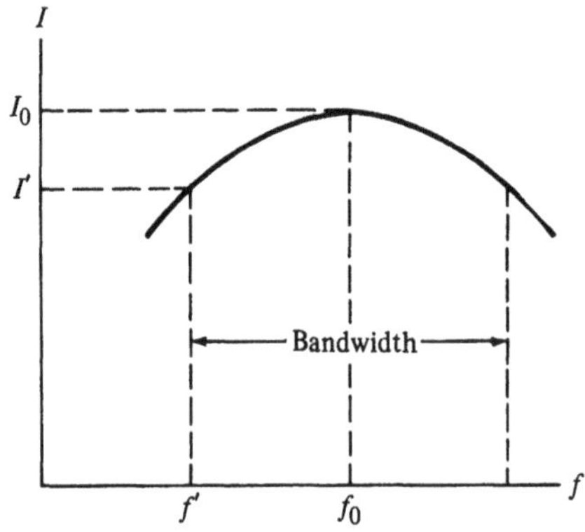

For half power,

$$EI'\cos\theta = \frac{EI_0}{2}$$

or

$$EI_0\cos^2\theta = \frac{EI_0}{2}.$$

But

$$\cos^2\theta = \tfrac{1}{2},$$

So

$$\cos\theta = 1/\sqrt{2} = 0.707$$
$$\theta = 45°.$$

At a power factor of 0.707,

$$R = X_L - X_C.$$

This resistance will produce a half-power bandwidth of $2f'$.

PROBLEMS

1. What resistance is required in the circuit shown below to produce a resonant frequency of 1000 Hz with a half-power bandwidth of 100 Hz?

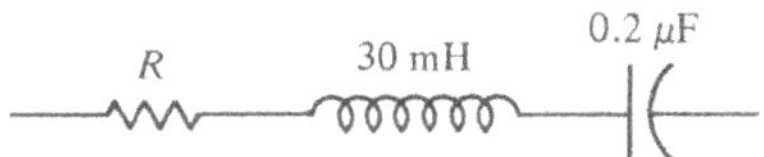

a. 5230 Ω.
b. 714 Ω.
c. 4750 Ω.
d. 659 Ω.
e. 438 Ω.

2. The natural frequency of the following circuit is:

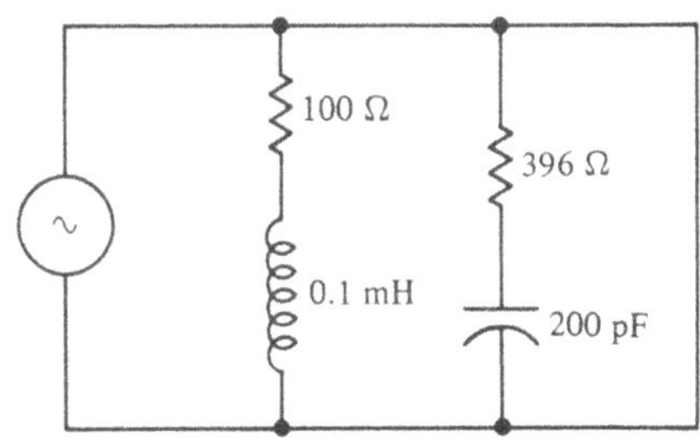

a. 1.13 MHz.
b. 2.62 GHz.
c. 468 kHz.
d. 1100 Hz.
e. Resonance does not occur.

Check your answers.

Answers

1. d.
2. e.

N. AFTERNOON PROBLEM SET

Examine the following circuit:

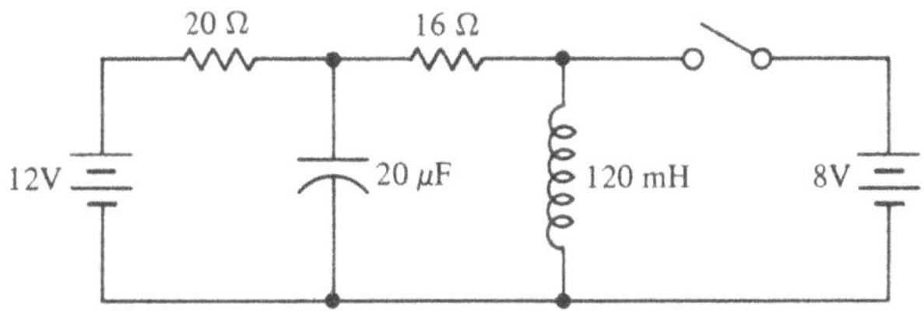

1. The circuit is at steady state when the switch is closed. What is the current through the 12-V battery just after the switch closes?

a. 2 A.
b. 1.6 A.
c. 0.33 A.
d. 0.25 A.
e. 3.6 A.

2. What is the current through the 8-V battery just after the switch closes?

a. 1 A.
b. 1.6 A.
c. 0.8 A.
d. 0.5 A.
e. 0.33 A.

3. Assume that the circuit elements are unknown, the switch remains open, and the 12-V battery is replaced with a 12-V alternator. In the left-hand circuit current equals 1 A and power equals 10 W. What is the total resistance in the circuit?

a. 8 Ω.
b. 10 Ω.
c. 12 Ω.
d. 16 Ω.
e. 28 Ω.

4. With the circuit described in question 3 above, what is the total reactance in the circuit?

a. 5.2 Ω.
b. 4.8 Ω.
c. 8.7 Ω.
d. 12.6 Ω.
e. 6.6 Ω.

5. As alternator frequency is increased, current increases. Reactance is:

a. Capacitive.
b. Inductive.
c. Capacitive and inductive.
d. Zero.
e. None of the above.

6. Assume that the circuit elements are unknown except that the inductor is open and that the left alternator has an unknown voltage but operates at 60 Hz. The total voltage drop across the resistors is 5 V and across the capacitor 5 V. What is the voltage of the alternator?

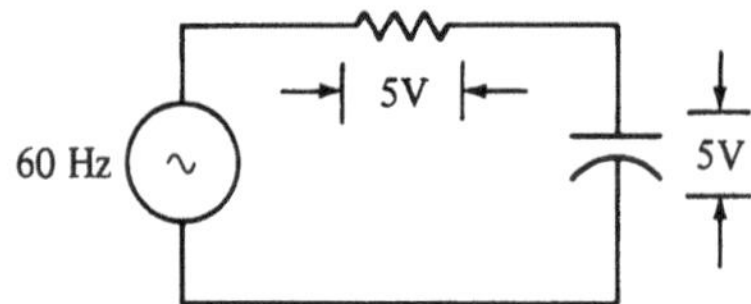

a. 5 V.
b. 6 V.
c. 7 V.
d. 8 V.
e. 9 V.

7. What is the power factor in the circuit described in question 6 above?

a. 0.707 leading.
b. 0.707 lagging.
c. 0.866 leading.
d. 0.866 lagging.
e. None of the above.

8. The circuit is changed as follows:

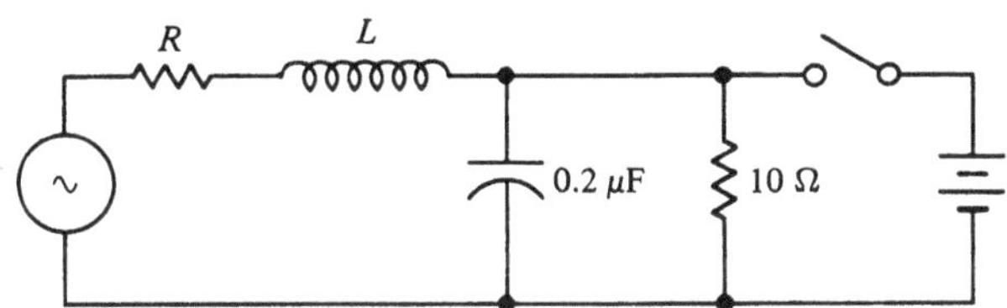

It is found that the resonant frequency of the left-hand circuit is 2000 Hz. What is the inductive reactance at that frequency?

a. 436 Ω.
b. 128 Ω.
c. 1364 Ω.
d. 398 Ω.
e. 532 Ω.

9. With the conditions of question 8 above, what is the inductance?

a. 26.4 mH.
b. 31.6 mH.
c. 16.3 mH.
d. 8.4 mH.
e. 64.2 mH.

10. If the half-power bandwidth is to be 100 Hz, what is the closest value of the resistor?

a. 10 Ω.
b. 15 Ω.
c. 20 Ω.
d. 25 Ω.
e. 30 Ω.

Check your answers.

Answers

1. c.
2. d.
3. b.
4. e.
5. a.
6. c.
7. a.
8. d.
9. b.
10. c.

18 Engineering Economics

Discussion of and problems related to costs and revenue, depreciation, time value of money, payments and annuities, and probabilistic costs and payments.

A. COSTS AND REVENUE

Engineering economics as defined by the Engineering Fundamentals Examination is most nearly equivalent to the academic subject of cost accounting. Throughout this chapter the viewpoint will be that of an organization's manager who wishes to make engineering decisions best suited to the organization's goals. The "best" measure of performance in business is usually money. Hence, a primary performance measurement is the cost and revenue situation for a particular organization.

Elements of Cost

Fixed costs (in a manufacturing situation) are costs accrued prior to the production of the first item. They are capital expenditures which cannot be recovered later, e.g., set-up and tear-down costs, tools and tooling only applicable to a specific job, or special purpose machines and equipment.

Variable costs (again in a manufacturing situation) are costs which accrue in direct proportion to the number of items produced, e.g., direct labor, direct material, depreciation, certain supplies, and other items of manufacturing expense.

Semi-variable costs are costs which remain fixed over a short period of production output but increase in systematic steps if the production output is increased sufficiently. Graphically:

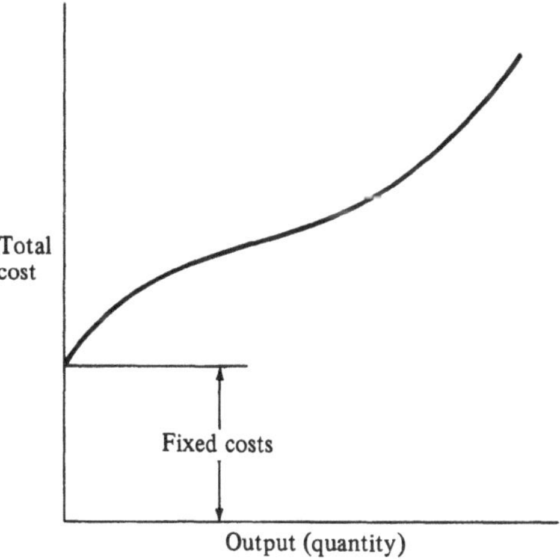

Revenue

Revenue is income derived from sales. Graphically:

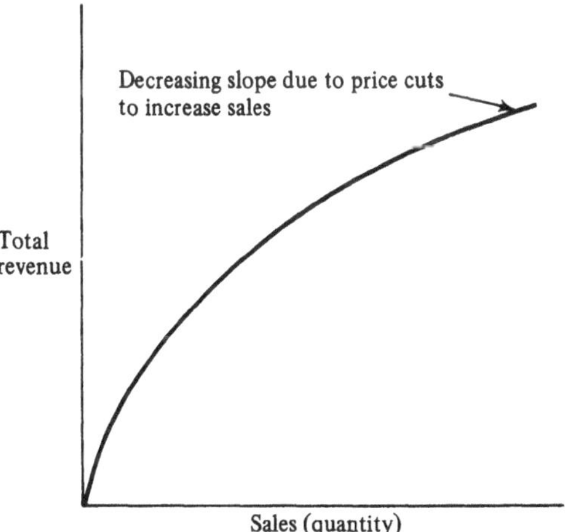

Since the above curves are empirical, and since precise data is often not available, the curves are often approximated by straight lines.

Breakeven Analysis

The breakeven point is that point of production where revenues equal costs. Graphically:

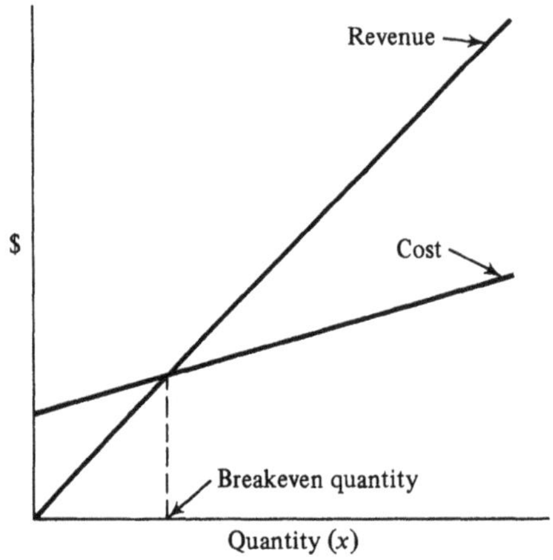

Profit Maximization

Profit is revenue less cost. If the revenue and cost curves are second order or higher polynomials, a certain output quantity maximizes profit. Graphically:

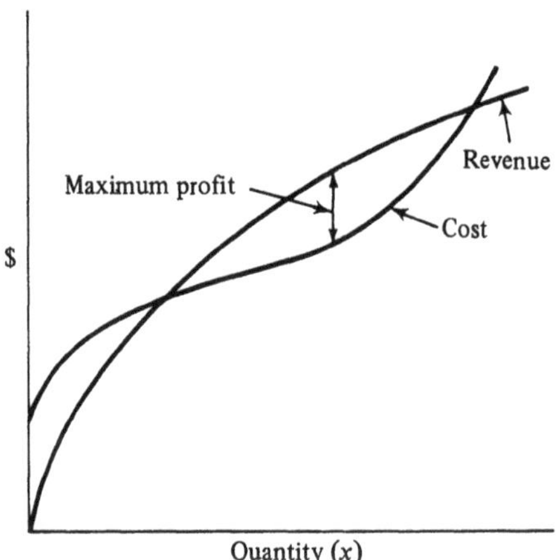

Cost Minimization

Unit costs will be at a minimum at a certain output quantity (not necessarily the maximum-profit quantity). To obtain unit costs, divide the total costs by the number of units.

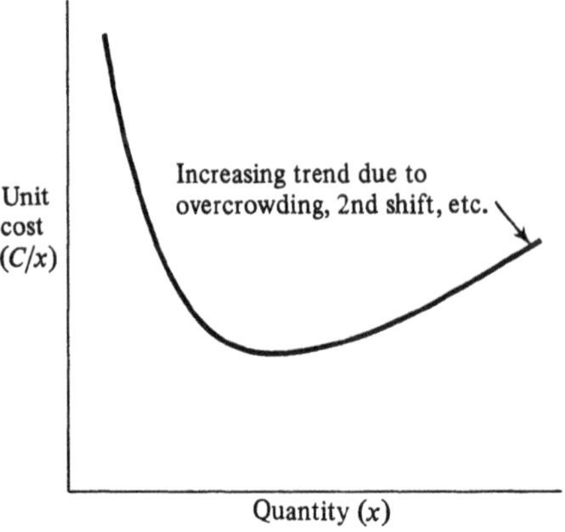

Costs and Revenue:
$C = f(x)$
$R = f(x)$
$\text{Profit} = R - C$
$\text{Unit costs} = C/x.$

Example

With the cost and revenue curves given below, determine fixed costs, the breakeven point, the output leading to, and the amount of, maximum profit.

$$R = 145x - 10x^2$$

$$C = \frac{x^3}{3} + 65x - 8x^2 + 260$$

$$FC = 260 \text{ (not dependent on } x\text{)}.$$

At the breakeven point:

$$C = R$$

$$145x - 10x^2 = \frac{x^3}{3} + 65X - 8x^2 + 260$$

$$x = 4.2 \text{ units of output at breakeven.}$$

Maximize profit:

$$P = R - C = \frac{-x^3}{3} - 2x^2 + 80x - 260.$$

Take the first derivative and set it equal to zero:

$$\frac{dp}{dx} = -x^2 - 4x + 80 = 0$$

$$x = 7.$$

Hence profit will be maximized at an output of 7 units. The amount of profit can be calculated by substituting $x = 7$ in the equation $P = R - C$.

Minimize costs:

$$\text{Unit cost is } \frac{C}{x} = \frac{x^2}{3} + 65 - 8x + \frac{260}{x}.$$

Minimum cost is at the output where

$$\frac{d(C/x)}{dx} = 0 = \frac{2x}{3} - 8 - \frac{260}{x^2}$$

or where

$$x = 14 \text{ units.}$$

PROBLEM

The cost of hand-wiring a control console is \$600/console. This cost can be eliminated by using an integrated circuit which costs \$100/console. The cost of designing the circuit is \$5,000. If a firm requires a one-year payback, what sales forecast will justify this design change?

a. 25 units.
b. 5 units.
c. 100 units.
d. 10 units.
e. 125 units.

Check your answer.

Answer

d.

B. DEPRECIATION

Depreciation of equipment is one element of fixed (or sometimes semi-variable) costs. Depreciation is the reduction in value of property due to its decreased ability to perform present and future service.

Depreciation is an accounting technique to reduce the value of a capital asset on a firm's annual report. Depreciation more accurately reports a firm's net worth when assets have a finite useful life. Further, depreciation allows a certain portion of an asset to be charged to the annual expense of doing business, thus reducing taxable profit and income tax.

Depreciation does not necessarily reflect the actual market value at any given point in time. Rather it is a systematic way of writing off an asset which has the sanction of the stockholders and the Internal Revenue Service.

Actual depreciation is the true decrease in value as determined by present market value; theoretical depreciation is an estimate of the actual depreciation. Methods used to determine theoretical depreciation include:

- straight-line depreciation,
- fixed percentage of diminishing balance (declining balance), and
- sum-of-the-years'-digits method.

Straight-line Depreciation

Annual depreciation (straight-line) is the depreciable value divided by the number of years of useful life. For example, a machine which costs \$1,200 new is worth only \$200 at the end of ten years. The annual depreciation is

$$D = \frac{\$1200 - \$200}{10 \text{ years}} = \$100.$$

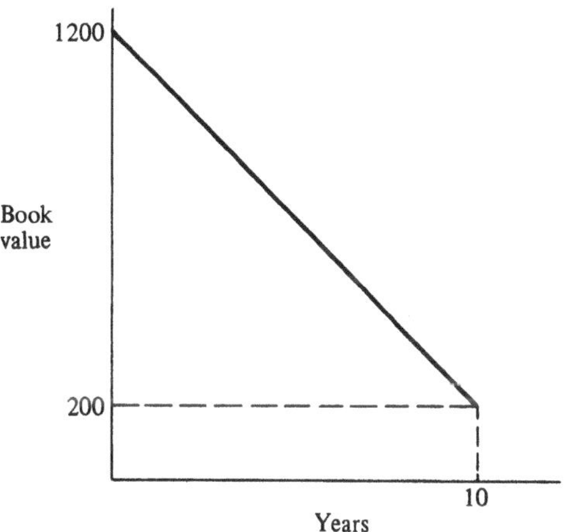

Declining Balance Depreciation

This is an accelerated depreciation technique which affords the following advantages:

- better reflecting market value on equipment with a high probability of early technological obsolescence, and
- deferring income taxes to later years.

Annual depreciation is equal to a constant percentage (twice the appropriate straight-line rate—called double declining balance) of whatever undepreciated balance is left at the beginning of that year.

In the example above:

1st year depreciation	$D_1 = (.20)(1000) = \$200$
2nd year depreciation	$D_2 = (.20)(800) = \$160$

This is known as an accelerated depreciation because the rate is higher in early years.

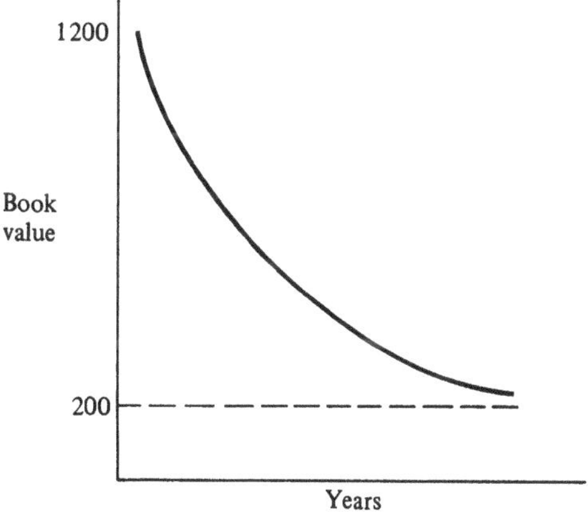

Sum-of-the-years'-digits Depreciation

With this method, sum the number of years of useful life. In the example above (10 years):

$$1 + 2 + \cdots + 10 = 55.$$

Each year's annual depreciation is based on the remaining years of useful life divided by this sum.

$$\text{1st year depreciation} \quad D_1 = \frac{10}{55}(1000) = \$181.82.$$

$$\text{2nd year depreciation} \quad D_2 = \frac{9}{55}(1000) = \$163.64.$$

This is also an accelerated depreciation scheme, although not as accelerated as declining balance.

In both the declining balance method and the sum-of-the-years' digits method it is conventional to switch to a straight line rate in later years.

Depreciation:

Straight-line:

$$\text{annual depreciation} = \frac{\text{total write-off}}{\text{number of years}}.$$

Declining Balance:

$$\text{annual depreciation} = \text{rate} \times \text{remaining book value}.$$

Sum-of-the-years'-digits:

$$\text{annual depreciation} = \frac{\text{year}}{\text{sum of years}} \times \text{total write-off}.$$

Example

A machine costs \$50,000 and has a scrap value of \$10,000 after ten years. It costs \$6,000 to maintain the machine, \$22,000 in wages to the operator, and \$1,000 for power to run it. The machine contributes \$50,000 to net earnings. At a tax rate of 50% and with straight-line depreciation, what is the profit generated by this machine?

Revenues	\$50,000	
less costs:		
Maintenance		\$ 6,000
Wages		22,000
Power		1,000
Depreciation		4,000
		33,000
Pretax profit	\$17,000	
Less tax	8,500	
Profit	\$ 8,500	

PROBLEMS

1. Which of the following is *not* a consideration in selecting a depreciation technique?

   a. Tax deferment.
   b. Accepted accounting practices.
   c. Profit maximization.
   d. Cost minimization.
   e. Technological obsolescence.

2. A machine costs \$10,000. The entire amount is to be written off in ten years. Income tax is 50%. How much will be saved in the third year by selecting sum-of-the-years'-digits method over straight-line depreciation?

   a. \$1455
   b. \$227
   c. \$373
   d. \$846
   e. \$1255

Check your answers.

Answers

1. d.
2. b.

C. TIME VALUE OF MONEY

When a decision is made to invest money in a piece of capital equipment, the equipment should yield a return. There is always the alternative of not buying the equipment and placing the money at interest instead. If the return offered by the equipment is less than the return from interest, then the equipment is uneconomical. This leads to calculations of return on investment.

Notation

P = present worth of an investment, also initial cost. The value of money in hand today.
F = future value, present worth plus accrued interest. The amount of money to be paid or received at some time in the future.
n = number of time periods, usually years, but could be months, quarters, etc.
i = periodic interest rate ($0 < i < 1$). The period must correspond to the units of n.

If P is placed in the bank today at an annual interest rate i and left to accumulate compounded interest for n years, at the end of n years the amount in the account will equal F.

Compound Interest

In the illustration above, the future value F is related to the present value P by the following formula:

$$F_n = P(1+i)^n,$$

or, rearranging,

$$P = F_n(1+i)^{-n}.$$

The terms $(1+i)^n$ and $(1+i)^{-n}$ are called *compound amount factor* and *present value factor* respectively. They can be evaluated by one of the following means:

- interest tables,
- electronic calculator, or
- logarithms.

Future value:

$$F_n = P(1+i)^n = (F/P, i, n).$$

Present value:

$$P = F_n(1+i)^{-n} = (P/F, i, n).$$

Example A

$10,000 invested at 6%/annum for 10 years will yield

$$\begin{aligned} F_n &= P(1+i)^n \\ F_{10} &= 10{,}000(1+0.06)^{10} \\ &= 10{,}000(1.7908) \\ &= \$17{,}908. \end{aligned}$$

Example B

We wish to determine which of two machines to purchase. Both have equal capacity and operating costs. Machine A costs $12,000 and has a scrap value of $2,000 after 10 years. Machine B costs $11,000 but is worthless after 10 years. Money is available to the firm at 5%/annum.

This decision can be made by present-value analysis:

$$\begin{aligned} P_A &= 12{,}000 - 2{,}000(0.61391) \\ &= \$10{,}780 \\ P_B &= \$11{,}000 \end{aligned}$$

Decision: Buy Machine A. (This problem could also have been solved by comparing future values.)

PROBLEMS

1. The bank uses the following formula to compound interest in a passbook savings account:

$$F = P\left(1 + \frac{i}{4}\right)^{4n}.$$

Interest is stated as an annual rate. How are they compounding?

a. Daily.
b. Weekly.
c. Monthly.
d. Quarterly.
e. Annually.

2. In a passbook savings account with monthly compounding and 6% per annum, your money will increase by half in:

a. 5 years.
b. 7 years.
c. 9 years.
d. 11 years.
e. 13 years.

Check your answers.

Answers

1. d.
2. b.

D. PAYMENTS AND ANNUITIES

A periodic payment or annuity A can be related to either present value P or future value F by the following formulas:

$$F_n = A\left[\frac{(1+i)^n - 1}{i}\right]$$

$$P = A\left[\frac{1-(1+i)^{-n}}{i}\right].$$

Again, tables are available for the above two factors.

Payments into a fund designed to have a certain future value constitute a "sinking fund" and are used to offset known future obligations.

Annuities in Perpetuity

In certain long-lived capital investments such as public works programs, derived benefits are assumed to continue forever. In other words, in the preceding formulas $n = \infty$. With this substitution, the present value formula becomes:

$$P = A\left[\frac{1-(1+i)^{-\infty}}{i}\right]$$

$$= A\left[\frac{1}{i} - \frac{1}{i(1+i)^{\infty}}\right]$$

$$= \frac{A}{i}.$$

Future value of a series of payments:

$$F_n = A\left[\frac{(1+i)^n - 1}{i}\right] = (F/A, i, n).$$

Present value of a series of payments:

$$P = A\left[\frac{1-(1+i)^{-n}}{i}\right] = (P/A, i, n).$$

Example A

A firm's criteria for capital investments is a return on investment of at least 15%. A \$100,000 machine with a useful life of 12 years is under consideration. It is estimated that its quarterly contribution to net income will be \$5,500. Should the firm purchase the machine?

$$100{,}000 = 5{,}500\,\frac{1-(1+i)^{-48}}{i}.$$

By trial and error, using the tables:

$$i = 5\%/\text{quarter}$$

$$= 20\%/\text{year}.$$

Decision: Buy the machine.

Example B

Annual maintenance costs for a particular section of highway pavement are \$2,000. The placement of a new surface would reduce the annual maintenance cost to \$500 per year for the first 5 years and to \$1000 per year for the next 5 years. The annual maintenance after 10 years would again be \$2000. If maintenance costs are the only saving, what maximum investment can be justified for the new surface? Assume interest at 4%.

The benefits are:

$1,500/year for the first 5 years, and

$1,000/year for the next 5 years.

What present value is equivalent to this stream of savings if $i = 4\%$?

This can be considered as $1,000/year for 10 years, plus an additional savings of $5,000/year for the first 5 years.

$$P = (1{,}000)(8.111) + (500)(4.452)$$

$$= \$10{,}337.$$

Conclusion: Investment of $10,337.

Example C

A dam was constructed for $200,000. The annual maintenance cost is $5,000, which is in effect an annuity in perpetuity. If interest is at 5%, what is the capitalized cost of the dam including maintenance?

Capitalized cost is defined as the present worth of all costs including perpetual service and is generally used in connection with public works projects. In this situation $n = \infty$.

$$\text{Capitalized cost} = \$200{,}000 + \frac{R}{i} = \$200{,}000 + \frac{\$5{,}000}{0.05} = \$300{,}000.$$

PROBLEMS

1. A 40-year-old inventor developed a carburetor which will allow a car to achieve 100 miles per gallon. He is entertaining the following offers made by various automobile manufacturers. Which offer should he accept? (Disregard any tax implications.)

   a. $80,000 in cash.
   b. A royalty of 6% on sales of $140,000 for the 10 year life of the patent.
   c. A 20-year annuity of $5,000 per year (money is worth 8%).
   d. A retirement annuity of $10,000 per year beginning at age 60 (he expects to live to age 80).
   e. Any of the above since they are all essentially equal.

2. A new vertical mill for a tool-and-die shop costs $7,000 and is expected to last 15 years. At the end of this time it can be sold as salvage for $1,000. The extra taxes and insurance for this mill are $300 per year. It is expected that the average cost of maintenance will be $20 per month. This firm uses straight-line depreciation and money is available at 8%. The annual cost of the mill is:

   a. $1084.
   b. $940.
   c. $1276.
   d. $1260.
   e. $1180.

Check your answers.

Answers

1. d.
2. c.
   Use average interest.

E. PROBABILISTIC COSTS AND PAYMENTS

Since the economic future is often uncertain, the gambling concept of "expected value" is used in economic decisions. In gambling, the expected value is the fair cost of playing a game. It is the reward multiplied by the probability of winning. In economics, the expected value is the probabilistic cost or payment multiplied by the probability that it will occur.

> Expected Value:
>
> $$EV = (\text{cost or payment})(\text{probability}).$$

Example

A man buys a lawn mower for \$100. Its average life is 5 years, but it is likely to fail completely at any time during those five years. What annual cost should he use in an economic analysis?

In any given year the annual cost is the replacement cost times the probability that it will have to be replaced:

$$\text{Cost} = (100)(\tfrac{1}{5}) = \$20/\text{year}.$$

These costs as well as the probabilities are mutually exclusive, i.e., he will have to replace the mower in the first year or the second year or the third year, etc.

PROBLEM

A radio antenna is to be constructed in an earthquake zone. It will last indefinitely, but it will not withstand an earthquake. Seismologists say that earthquake probability follows an approximate cycle. Their estimate of the probabilities of an earthquake are as follows:

15 years from now	0.05
16 years from now	0.25
17 years from now	0.40
18 years from now	0.25
19 years from now	0.05

The need for the antenna will exist for 25 years. Money costs 8%. The cost of building the antenna is \$50,000. The capitalized cost of the antenna is:

a. \$63,549.
b. \$62,510.

c. \$63,256.
d. \$50,000.
e. \$100,000.

Check your answer.

Answer

a.
The capitalized cost is the present value of all costs present and future.

F. AFTERNOON PROBLEM SET

The following two punch presses are under consideration in a metal fabricating shop:

	Johnson Model S	*AJAX Speedipunch*
1st cost	\$150,000	\$250,000
Life	10 years	15 years
Maintenance	\$1,000/year	\$500/year for 1st 10 years increasing by \$100/year for each year thereafter
Salvage	\$10,000	\$15,000

1. At an interest rate of 8%, which machine has a present value advantage and approximately how much?

   a. Johnson, \$50,000.
   b. Johnson, \$100,000.
   c. AJAX, \$80,000.
   d. AJAX, \$30,000.
   e. Both are equal.

2. What is the annual cost for the Johnson machine using the capital recovery method?

   a. \$22,450.
   b. \$22,660.
   c. \$27,150.
   d. \$28,050.
   e. \$29,200.

3. What is the annual cost for the Johnson machine using straight-line depreciation + interest?

   a. \$20,040.
   b. \$20,542.
   c. \$21,960.
   d. \$24,640.
   e. \$26,440.

4. Which of the following costs would be used for income tax purposes?

   a. Annual maintenance.
   b. Depreciation + interest.
   c. Capital recovery.
   d. a and c.
   e. a and b.

5. If straight-line depreciation is used and the tax rate is 50%, what is the effective present value of the Johnson machine?

   a. $152,000.
   b. $96,000.
   c. $132,000.
   d. $105,000.
   e. $84,000.

6. It is expected that technological obsolescence will reduce the value of the Johnson machine to $50,000 after 5 years. What declining-balance rate would make the balance sheet reflect this?

   a. 5%.
   b. 10%.
   c. 15%.
   d. 20%.
   e. 25%.

7. The third-year depreciation of the AJAX machine using sum-of-the-years'-digits is approximately:

   a. $25,000.
   b. $25,500.
   c. $26,000.
   d. $26,500.
   e. $27,000.

8. What is the present value of the tax savings over the life of the machine using the method above as opposed to straight-line depreciation?

   a. $78,800.
   b. $82,400.
   c. $89,600.
   d. $90,500.
   e. $96,200.

9. In a given year the Johnson machine has fixed costs of $15,000 and variable costs of $100 per piece part. What is the breakeven quantity if the parts sell for $150?

   a. 100.
   b. 200.
   c. 300.
   d. 400.
   e. 500.

10. An automatic oiler is available for the AJAX press which will reduce the maintenance cost in the last five years by $100 per year. What is it worth as an option on the machine when purchased?

    a. $185.
    b. $400.
    c. $216.
    d. $135.
    e. $375.

Check your answers.

Answers

1. b.
2. b.
3. c.
4. e.
5. d.
6. d.
7. b.
8. a.
9. c.
10. a.

A FINAL WORD

This book combines the efforts of several years of helping engineers prepare for the National Engineering Fundamentals Examination. Experience has shown that the basic materials covered in this book will correspond to the major portion of the material covered in the examination. After using this book, you will enter the examination with a proper amount of drill in the basic engineering disciplines and recent practice in augmenting your knowledge with texts and handbooks. You probably noticed that some necessary information was *not* included in the text. This was done purposely to encourage you to refer to reference material that may be useful during the examination.

Now that you have completed this programmed review, you should be ready for the examination. The following suggestions might be of help in the exam:

- If your state, like most, has an open-book exam, take with you this text and all the reference materials you used to augment it.
- Get a good night's sleep before the exam. Know the parking arrangements and the location of the examining room. You don't want to be late.
- Take a slide rule, calculator, and any other implements you used in preparing for the exam. If you just bought a new calculator, be sure you are familiar with it and that the batteries are strong. Be sure to have three or four sharpened pencils with good erasers with you.
- The directions for taking the exam are a bit complex for someone working under pressure. Be sure you understand all directions *before* you start.
- The time pressure in the morning session of the exam is great. To obtain the maximum score, go through all the short multiple-choice problems, answering *only* those problems you know you can answer quickly. Go through the test a second time, working the slightly more difficult ones. Don't be dismayed if you don't finish in the morning. You probably wouldn't have answered correctly those problems which you skipped.
- Don't decide in advance to skip certain areas. Although you may be a mechanical engineer, there may be some easy electrical problems. Why throw these points away?

The time pressure is much less in the afternoon; you have four hours in which to complete five problems each consisting of ten multiple-choice questions. If you are properly prepared, you will have ample time to plot a strategy. Read every problem. Select the five problems you are going to solve. Begin with the easiest and work through to the most difficult. You will probably be able to work two or three problems in twenty minutes each, or less. You will then have time to research the remaining two or three problems using the reference materials you brought.

The examination is a very exhausting ordeal. Commonly when examinees leave the exam, they are not overly optimistic about the results. Don't be despondent. If you were well prepared and used your examination time wisely, you should pass.

The authors wish you luck and look forward to welcoming you into the profession of engineering.

Index

INDEX

www.ingramcontent.com/pod-product-compliance
Ingram Content Group UK Ltd.
Pitfield, Milton Keynes, MK11 3LW, UK
UKHW061831190726
13855UKWH00005B/1749

* 9 7 8 1 4 7 5 7 1 2 2 4 7 *